Development and Control of Medicines and Medical Devices

Development and Control of Medicines and Medical Devices

Robin J Harman
BPharm, PhD, MRPharmS
Independent Pharmaceutical and Regulatory Consultant
Farnham, Surrey, UK

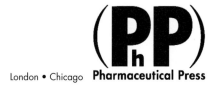

London • Chicago **Pharmaceutical Press**

Published by the Pharmaceutical Press
Publications division of the Royal Pharmaceutical Society of Great Britain

1 Lambeth High Street, London SE1 7JN, UK
100 South Atkinson Road. Suite 206, Grayslake, IL 60030-7820, USA

© Pharmaceutical Press 2004

(PP) is a trade mark of Pharmaceutical Press

First published 2004

Text design by Barker/Hilson, Lyme Regis, Dorset
Typeset by Gray Publishing, Tunbridge Wells, Kent
Printed in Great Britain by TJ International, Padstow, Cornwall

ISBN 0 85369 567 9

All rights reserved. No part of this publication may be reproduced, stored in a retrieval system, or transmitted in any form or by any means, without the prior written permission of the copyright holder.
 The publisher makes no representation, express or implied, with regard to the accuracy of the information contained in this book and cannot accept any legal responsibility or liability for any errors or omissions that may be made.

A catalogue record for this book is available from the British Library

Contents

Preface vii
About the author xiii

Part A

Developing medicines and medical devices

1	Introduction to the drug development process	3
2	Options in the registration of medicinal products	15
3	Quality issues	29
4	Pharmacotoxicological studies	59
5	Clinical studies	89
6	Pharmacovigilance	127
7	Medical devices and their control	141
8	Ethical issues	147

Part B

Organisations controlling medicines and medical devices

9	MHRA – Medicinal products	157
10	MHRA – Medical devices	171
11	The EMEA – Supranational drug regulation	179
12	The National Institute for Clinical Excellence	195
13	International perspectives	215

Appendices

Appendix 1 EU regulatory authorities	229
Appendix 2 WMA Declaration of Helsinki	233
Appendix 3 WHO member states by region	239

Index 243

Preface

When looking at a tablet or a capsule, it is hard to reconcile its visual simplicity with the many-layered and highly complex process that has led to its presence in your hand ready for administration.

Nevertheless, that process by which a chemical or biological agent is transformed into a medicinal product that can be easily and safely used is extremely complex, lengthy and expensive. Equally, manufacturers of medicinal products operate in perhaps one of the most regulated of commercial environments. Considerable – and in no way guaranteed – investment must be made prior to authorisation being given to market a product and to achieve any return on that investment.

This book describes the three primary hurdles that must be overcome for a medicinal product to be allowed to be marketed: that a medicinal product must be of acceptable quality, safety and efficacy. It also more briefly reviews the parallel processes that must be undertaken by manufacturers of medical devices, who must ensure that their products are both of acceptable quality and effective in their intended purpose.

It is often easy to forget that almost all of the medicinal products now available have been developed during the last 50 years, with by far the most effective having been produced within the most recent 20 years. Before the 1950s, the range of available therapeutically proven tools was paltry. Even by the end of the 1950s, the only significant advances were the use of cortisone in rheumatoid arthritis and of imipramine in the treatment of depression.

It was the 1960s that heralded the first major therapeutic revolution, which included the development of metronidazole in 1960, allopurinol in 1961, the first oral contraceptives in 1962, and ampicillin in 1963. (The dates of introduction of some other major products from 1960 to 1990 are shown in Table P.1.)

Equally importantly for the control of the development of medicines was the realisation in 1962 that thalidomide taken by pregnant women caused bilateral limb reductions (e.g. amelia and phocomelia) due to its effects on fetal organ development. Thalidomide had been introduced in 1956 as a sedative and a remedy for influenza, and its use highlighted the inadequacy of the testing (and especially the toxicological assessment) undertaken prior to launching new products. Most agents that produced

Table P.1 Launch dates of some major pharmaceutical products 1960–1990[1]

Year	Product	Initial use
1962	Azathioprine	Immunosuppression
1964	Ibuprofen/flurbiprofen	Arthritis and inflammation
1965	Propranolol	Antihypertensive
1967	Beclometasone	Asthma
1968	Sodium cromoglicate	Asthma
1969	Salbutamol	Asthma
1970	Levodopa	Parkinson's disease
1973	Tamoxifen	Hormone-dependent tumours
1975	Clotrimazole	Fungal infections
1976	Cimetidine	Peptic ulceration
1978	Ranitidine	Peptic ulceration
1981	Captopril	Antihypertensive
1982	Fluconazole	Fungal infections
1983	Sumatriptan	Migraine
1985	Aciclovir	Herpes infections
1986	Orthoclone	For organ transplantation
1987	Zidovudine	Treatment of AIDS
1988	Diclofenac	Anti-inflammatory agent
1989	Simvastatin	Lipid-lowering agent

such devastating effects would also cause the fetus to be aborted; the difference with thalidomide was that the pregnancies went to full term, producing grossly physically disabled individuals who were otherwise relatively healthy.

Many countries acted following the thalidomide catastrophe to tighten up the controls on the development and introduction of new medicines. In the European Economic Community, then with six Member States, the first major piece of pharmaceutical legislation, Directive 65/65/EEC, was the outcome; in the UK, it was the Medicines Act 1968.

Since that time, statutory controls have extended into almost every facet of the programme to develop new medicinal agents: from the design of the tests to ensure the stability of the active ingredient and the final formulated product; through the conduct of clinical trials and the protection of human subjects; to the increasingly stringent requirements for monitoring the performance of products after a marketing authorisation has been granted and the product is more widely used in the general population. It is not only the development process that is closely regulated. All aspects of the advertising of prescription-only medicines to the medical profession and of nonprescription medicines to the general public are also closely controlled. The design of packaging and the information provided by the manufacturer to the user of the medicine also have to be approved prior to their use.

With the ever-increasing volume of regulations, the investment required to develop a medicinal product has continued to increase. The pan-

European trade association for the pharmaceutical industry, the European Federation of Pharmaceutical Industries and Associations (EFPIA), has estimated the cost in 2002 of developing a new chemical or biological entity to be almost €900 million (about £630 million).[2]

This increasing cost has to be balanced against the ongoing trend of governments to exert continual downward pressure on funds available for healthcare in individual countries. Many countries now routinely carry out health technology assessments. In these, the value of a new medicinal product is assessed against other forms of treatment already available and, if it is deemed not to provide significantly enhanced benefit, reimbursement of the cost of the medicine may not be permitted. The considerable investment by the manufacturer can easily be rendered nonreturnable in such a decision-making process.

This book therefore looks at the two major aspects of the development of medicines and medical devices: the research and development procedures which have to be completed prior to being allowed to market the product; and the organisations and processes which control and regulate those procedures. The emphasis is primarily on the systems and controls that operate in the UK; as these are based on European legislation, much of what is described, especially with regard to the development procedures, is also applicable across all 25 Member States of the EU.

Chapter 1 provides an introduction to the drug research and development process and the ways in which its efficiency can be maximised. A summary of the overall drug development programme is provided, and the pharmaceutical studies, preclinical toxicological studies, clinical studies and post-marketing programme required for all new medicinal products are described. The tremendously high attrition rate for newly synthesised chemicals as each of these phases of development is reached reflects the complexity of the testing that must be undertaken and the very stringent limitations placed upon the overall process.

The options for approval of a medicinal product, and the way in which legislative controls have developed in the UK, are described in Chapter 2, which also summarises the most important legislation that has been passed since that first European Directive 65/65/EEC. The development of a single EU marketing authorisation is also explained, together with the creation of the first pan-European regulatory authority, the European Agency for the Evaluation of Medicinal Products (EMEA). The most recent changes to European procedures, encompassing the format of the Common Technical Document and the ongoing review of EU pharmaceutical legislation, are also described.

Chapters 3, 4 and 5 explain the detailed requirements of the testing that has to be undertaken to generate the data required to satisfy statutory controls in each of the criteria of quality, safety and efficacy. The data required range from the stability testing of active ingredients and finished products, through genotoxicity and mutagenicity testing, to clinical trials and the concept of good clinical practice. Every facet of the development process has come under statutory control. However, many of the requirements are laid down as guidance rather than being mandatory. This allows manufacturers a degree of flexibility in their development programmes, although any significant deviations from the guidance provided must be justified by the manufacturer in the submission to the regulatory authority.

Controls on medicinal products do not cease once an authorisation has been obtained – far from it. In many ways, the scope and range of reporting on the use of medicinal products has increased significantly over recent years. This has even led to the proposal that, if the reporting does not elicit any significant problems with the use of the product, the regular and in-depth reports may remove the need for the 5-yearly renewal process. Chapter 6 describes the pharmacovigilance requirements that must be fulfilled.

Most products used in the healthcare setting are classed not as medicinal products but as medical devices. A medical device can vary from a syringe to an operating table to a cardiac pacemaker. The legislation controlling the use of medical devices has developed separately from that governing pharmaceuticals, and Chapter 7 outlines current EU rules for general medical devices, active implantable medical devices and *in vitro* diagnostics. That classification of medical devices reflects the potential risks from their use and the degree of invasiveness into the body required in their use.

Chapter 8 considers some of the ethical issues affecting the use of healthcare products and their development. It must be remembered that all legislation for medicinal products and medical devices has evolved with the protection of public health as the primary concern. In developing such products, there exist equal demands for the health of those involved in clinical trials to be protected. It is a requirement of the ethical controls in drug development that none of the heinous crimes against the young and vulnerable practised in various conflicts around the world, especially in the twentieth century, are allowed to recur.

The second part of the book describes the roles of the organisations that exist to control the development of medicinal products and medical devices. Almost every country worldwide now has one or more of its own regulatory authorities. In some countries, there are separate organisations for human medicinal products, for veterinary medicinal products, and for medical devices. In others, one or more of these categories may be dealt with by a single organisation.

Chapters 9 and 10 describe the work of the UK regulatory authority, the Medicines and Healthcare products Regulatory Agency (MHRA). This deals with both medicinal products and medical devices, although they were dealt with by separate agencies prior to April 2003.

Medicinal products can also be approved for use in the UK by the EMEA, and its structure and functions are reviewed in Chapter 11. Created in 1995, it operates at a pan-European level, and carries out assessment of marketing authorisation applications which, if approved and issued by the European Commission, are valid throughout all EU Member States.

Chapter 12 explains the workings of the National Institute for Clinical Excellence (NICE), one of the first bodies created by government intended to add a degree of objectivity to the assessment and comparison of the clinical effectiveness and cost-effectiveness of new technologies with existing therapies. The guidance issued by NICE has been instrumental in limiting the availability of some new products because clinical effectiveness and cost-effectiveness have not been demonstrated. Equally, however, a positive assessment given by NICE ensures that the product is used throughout the NHS and can be highly beneficial to manufacturers.

It also has to be recognised that the pharmaceutical industry has long been global in its operations. Chapter 13 therefore reviews the ICH process (the International Conference on the Harmonisation of the Technical Requirements for the Registration of Pharmaceuticals for Human Use), in which regulators and the industry have worked together to try to reduce the costs to both parties of bringing new products to market. The structure and activities of the world's largest regulatory authority, the US Food and Drug Administration (FDA) are also briefly described. Outside the areas covered by the three major players in the pharmaceutical world (the EU, the USA and Japan), the role of the World Health Organization in ensuring that all countries are able to benefit from the development of new and improved healthcare products is also reviewed.

Some of these topics have been covered in articles published in the *Pharmaceutical Journal* over the last five years. However, all have required updating to reflect the ongoing changes in the regulatory framework that occur for all players in the exciting and challenging world of the development and control of medicines and medical devices.

References

1. Hall M, Kirkness B (eds). *An A to Z of British Medicines Research*, 2nd edn. London: Association of the British Pharmaceutical Industry, 1998.
2. European Commission. COM (2003) 383 final, Brussels, 01.07.2003: communication from the Commission to the Council, the European Parliament, the Economic and Social Committee and the Committee of the Regions: *A Stronger European-based Pharmaceutical Industry for the Benefit of the Patient – a Call for Action*. ISSN 02541475.

About the author

Robin J Harman PhD, MRPharmS has been an independent pharmaceutical and regulatory consultant, based in Farnham, Surrey, England, since 1998. He is co-editor of the second edition of the *Handbook of Pharmacy Healthcare* (Pharmaceutical Press, 2002); editor of the second edition of *Patient Care in Community Practice: a Handbook of Non-Medicinal Healthcare* (Pharmaceutical Press, 2002); and editor of the second edition of the *Handbook of Pharmacy Health Education* (Pharmaceutical Press, 2001).

He launched and was editor-in-chief of *The Regulatory Affairs Journal* and *The Regulatory Affairs Journal (Devices)* from 1990 to 1998, which continue to provide information to the pharmaceutical and medical devices industries, respectively. Previously, he was an editor in the Department of Pharmaceutical Sciences at the Royal Pharmaceutical Society of Great Britain. He edited the first edition of the *Handbook of Pharmacy Health-care: Diseases and Patient Advice* (Pharmaceutical Press, 1990), and authored the first edition of *Patient Care in Community Practice: a Handbook of Non-medicinal Health-care* (Pharmaceutical Press, 1989).

Part A

Developing medicines and medical devices

1

Introduction to the drug development process

The development of a medicinal product from a newly synthesised chemical compound, a chemical extracted from a naturally occurring source, or a compound produced by biotechnological processes is one of the most fascinating processes in which pharmacists can become involved. It challenges all presuppositions that one may have about the scientific aspects of pharmacy; and it makes use of the entire knowledge base that pharmacy undergraduates will have attained. Therefore, not only is being involved in the process an intellectually demanding, and hopefully satisfying, experience, it also brings together all the elements of a diverse and wide-ranging educational experience.

The only surprise about the drug development process in the pharmaceutical industry is the relatively small number of pharmacists who become actively involved in it. It is estimated that there are about 2000 pharmacists working in the pharmaceutical industry (i.e. about 5% of the total pharmacists on the Pharmaceutical Register).[1] Whilst pharmacists in the hospital service can also become involved in the process (e.g. the organisation of clinical trial materials), it is only within the pharmaceutical industry that pharmacists have the opportunity to become involved in several or all of the stages. Pharmacists in industry are actively involved in:

- basic synthetic chemical research
- pharmaceutical formulation development
- the manufacturing process
- toxicological studies
- all stages of clinical trials
- the regulatory affairs process, both in industry and in government regulatory authorities
- post-marketing surveillance, again both in industry and in government regulatory authorities
- sales, marketing and promotion of medicinal products
- medical information.

However, this book is not an advertisement for pharmacists to take full advantage of the opportunities that exist in the pharmaceutical industry. Rather, it is an exposition of the highly scientific and technical, and in many ways entrepreneurial, process that must take place to bring a new medicinal product to the marketplace and in which pharmacists can and do play an active and important part.

Creating the environment for efficient drug development

The drug development process is slow and very expensive, with high levels of drop-out of candidates. Of 10 000 molecules extracted, synthesised or tested, only one will usually traverse all the hurdles to become a newly authorised medicinal product. The entire process can take from 8 to 10 years for treatments for acute conditions, and up to 12 years for chronic illness treatments. The cost of the development process has to be borne before any revenue is earned from sales. This cost has been estimated to be about £630 million per new chemical entity. It is therefore vital that the research-based pharmaceutical industry has a healthy financial basis on which to be able to develop further new medicinal products. Various factors have been described as essential to the success of the research and development process:

- protection of intellectual property
- support of open vigorous competition
- favourable trade policies
- strong basic research infrastructure
- sufficient spending on secondary and tertiary education.[2]

In the USA, the amount spent by the research-based pharmaceutical industry on research and development was more than $20 billion in 1998, equivalent to 17% of US sales. The total global spend on research and development has been estimated to be $36 billion. However, it is suggested that investment alone is insufficient to produce innovation. Favourable national policies are also required, including:

- substantial government investment in basic biomedical research
- strong intellectual property protection
- free-market pricing for pharmaceuticals
- an efficient and transparent regulatory process
- access to global markets.[2]

The UK economic and business environment has proved particularly conducive to new medicinal product development. The UK is second only to the USA in the numbers of new medicinal products that have been developed, with six of the world's top 12 medicines developed in British laboratories.[3] One reason for this is that more than £8 million a day is spent on research and development by the UK pharmaceutical industry, amounting to an estimated £3 billion in 2001.[4] The industry spends by far the greatest amount of money each year on research and development of new medicinal products of all parties involved in contributing to health research costs:

- 70% is spent by the pharmaceutical industry
- 12% by medical research charities

- 10% by the Medical Research Council
- 4% by higher education institutions
- 2% by the UK Department of Health.[5]

The top ten pharmaceutical products in the UK in 2002 are listed in Table 1.1.

The stages in the discovery and development of a new medicinal product

There are many strands to the drug development process that must be followed simultaneously and coordinated effectively to maximise the return from the considerable financial investment. The importance of achieving this cannot be understated: doing so can represent the difference between having the market leader of a new therapeutic class of medicinal product and having the second member of the group, which will invariably be compared (often unfavourably) against the market leader. (This logic does not always apply. The first of the new group of H_2-receptor antagonists to reach the market, used to alleviate the symptoms of peptic ulcer, was cimetidine, for which SmithKline French (as it then was) was granted the first marketing authorisation in 1976. However, Glaxo produced its own new H_2-receptor antagonist, ranitidine, in 1978 and the Glaxo compound rapidly overtook cimetidine as the world's market leader and major money-earner.)

Table 1.1 Top UK pharmaceutical products 2002

Proprietary name	Drug name	Primary use	Manufacturer	Date of marketing authorisation	Total sales (£m)
Zocor	Simvastatin	Lipid regulator	MSD	May 89	310.67
Lipitor	Atorvastatin	Lipid regulator	Pfizer	Jan. 97	237.70
Zoton	Lansoprazole	Proton pump inhibitor for ulcer healing	Wyeth	Apr. 94	229.03
Istin	Amlodipine	Calcium channel blocker for hypertension and angina	Pfizer	Jan. 90	170.23
Losec	Omeprazole	Proton pump inhibitor for ulcer healing	AstraZeneca	Jun. 89	162.77
Zyprexa	Olanzapine	Schizophrenia	Eli Lilly	Oct. 96	121.07
Seretide	Fluticasone and salmeterol	Corticosteroid for chronic asthma	GlaxoSmithKline	Mar. 99	115.54
Lipostat	Pravastatin	Lipid regulator	Bristol Myers Squibb	Sept. 90	109.86
Tritace	Ramipril	Mild to moderate hypertension	Aventis	Mar. 90	104.33
Serevent	Salmeterol	Adrenoceptor agonist for chronic asthma	GlaxoSmithKline	Dec. 90	101.91

Based on information at www.abpi.org.uk/statistics,[4] source IMS, accessed February 2004.

One of the best guides to the stages of drug development is found in the two subvolumes of the *Notice to Applicants*. Produced by the European Commission, the *Notice to Applicants*, Volume 2A, covers procedures for obtaining a marketing authorisation; Volume 2B deals with the presentation and content of a marketing authorisation application (MAA). Both are part of the nine volumes of *The Rules Governing Medicinal Products in the European Union*, applicable in all 25 Member States of the European Union (EU) as the framework for assessing MAAs.[6] Although the nine volumes have no legal force, and any organisation submitting an MAA must follow the appropriate EU Regulations and Directives (or explain in detail any deviations from these legislative instruments), the texts are invaluable for compilation of MAAs and as a guide to the drug development process (see Table 1.2).

The development process can also be summarised in terms of the number of candidates that exist at each stage (Table 1.3).

Running in parallel to the above stages are chemical, biotechnological and pharmaceutical development procedures, preclinical toxicology, pharmacokinetic studies and long-term animal testing studies. Each of these areas is considered in detail in later chapters. A brief overview of the entire process is presented here.

Chemical, pharmaceutical and biological studies

Chemists and pharmacists in the pharmaceutical industry produce thousands of new compounds each year. No-one can predict which (if any) will successfully develop into a new medicinal product. All initial studies on a new compound are carried out *in vitro*; it is only much later in the development process that any *in vivo* testing is begun. A comprehensive profile of the new chemical is built up, including examination of its chemical stability, its ability to be prepared into various dosage forms (pharmaceutical development), and initial studies on its effects and its absorption, distribution, metabolism and excretion in animals (pharmacological studies and biological studies).

Chemical development

If initial pharmacological screening proves promising (i.e. if the compound has some or all of the pharmacological effects that might have been predicted from its chemical structure), compounds with minor variations on the chemical structure are usually prepared and also investigated. Do these structural changes improve the pharmacological profile (e.g. does a minor change in chemical structure produce higher animal blood levels)? Screening will also take place of unexpected effects that a chemical might have. It is vital at this early stage to maximise the potential of any chemical drug candidate: beneficial effects might lead to new avenues of research and development of other potential therapeutic benefits. Equally, more thorough testing of related compounds by a competitor could result in that competitor producing the market leader in a new therapeutic class.

Table 1.2 Presentation of the marketing authorisation application

The marketing authorisation application (MAA), which should be submitted in either a centralised procedure or a mutual recognition procedure, consists of administrative information and the necessary demonstration of quality, safety and efficacy of the product. (An explanation of the centralised and mutual recognition approval processes is given in Chapter 2.) This is presented in four Parts.

Part I Summary of the Dossier
Part IA	Administrative data
Part IB1	Summary of Product Characteristics (SPC)
Part IB2	Proposal for packaging, labelling and package insert
Part IB3	SPC already approved in the Member States
Part IC	Expert Reports
Part IC1	Expert Report on the chemical, pharmaceutical and biological documentation
Part IC2	Expert Report on the pharmacotoxicological (preclinical) documentation
Part IC3	Expert Report on the clinical documentation

Part II Chemical, pharmaceutical and biological documentation
Part IIA	Composition
Part IIB	Method of preparation
Part IIC	Control of starting materials
Part IID	Control tests on intermediate materials
Part IIE	Control tests on the finished product
Part IIF	Stability
Part IIG	Bioavailability/bioequivalence
Part IIH	Data related to the environment risk assessment for products containing GMOs (genetically modified organisms)
Part IIQ	Other information

Part III Pharmacotoxicological documentation
Part IIIA	Toxicity
Part IIIB	Reproductive function
Part IIIC	Embryo-fetal and perinatal toxicity
Part IIID	Mutagenic potential
Part IIIE	Carcinogenic potential
Part IIIF	Pharmacodynamics
Part IIIG	Pharmacokinetics
Part IIIH	Local tolerance
Part IIIQ	Other information
Part IIIR	Environment risk assessment

Part IV Clinical documentation
Part IVA	Clinical pharmacology
Part IVB	Clinical experience
Part IVQ	Other information

Table 1.3 Numbers of potential compounds at different stages of pharmaceutical research

Stage	No. of compounds
Basic research	Up to 10 000
Applied research	10–15
Clinical development	From 8 down to 1 by end
Regulatory assessment and approval	1
Post-marketing evaluation	1

Pharmacological screening

Many companies focus on specific therapeutic areas, either through historical precedent or because they have identified a particular therapeutic area as the most likely to produce chemicals of importance and with novel actions. The areas of research interest will also be in part determined by the current in-house scientific expertise.

Biotechnological screening

One of the major growth areas within the last 20 years has been the development of compounds derived from biotechnological processes. New companies involved specifically in biotechnology research have been formed; mainstream pharmaceutical companies have also diversified their research activities. A 1999 survey by US PhRMA (Pharmaceutical Research and Manufacturers of America)[7] found 350 new biotechnology medicines under development, with 140 pharmaceutical and biotechnology companies testing new products. At that time, the biotechnology revolution had already produced 54 new medicines; and 19 new biotechnology medicinal products were approved by the US Food and Drug Administration (FDA) between 1997 and 1999. The numbers have increased dramatically over the past 5 years.

The agents classed as biotechnological medicinal products include proteins, enzymes, antibodies, genetic materials and other naturally occurring substances that fight infection and disease. The production of biotechnological medicinal products is assisted by other living organisms: plant and animal cells, viruses and yeasts.

There are four primary areas in health care in which biotechnology research is being carried out: medicinal products, vaccines, diagnostic agents and gene therapy. Most medicinal products are proteins that normally occur naturally, including insulin products and human growth products. The US FDA and the European Agency for the Evaluation of Medicinal Products (EMEA) have approved biotechnological products for anaemia, cystic fibrosis, growth deficiency, hepatitis and transplant rejection.

A vaccine that has been developed to fight hepatitis B infection has the advantage over traditional vaccines of not requiring the presence of the actual virus (either live or attenuated) in the final product. Yeast cells and the inserted gene responsible for producing the hepatitis antigen are reproduced by a fermentation process similar to that used to produce beer. After purification, the hepatitis antigen stimulates the body's own production of anti-hepatitis antibodies.

Biotechnology diagnostic agents are used to detect a variety of diseases (e.g. to screen donated blood for human immunodeficiency virus (HIV) and hepatitis). Perhaps the most commonly used biotechnology diagnostic agent is the home pregnancy testing kit.

Hereditary genetic disorders have for a long time been untreatable by traditional chemotherapeutic agents. Now, a faulty or missing gene can be replaced by a biotechnologically produced gene. This technique has been used to treat, amongst other conditions, severe combined immunodeficiency disease, in which the body has no resistance to modern antigens.

Over one-third of the 350 new biotechnology medicines in development are for cancer (specifically melanoma, colorectal cancer, and prostatic and breast cancer). Among other diseases targeted by the 77 biotechnologically produced vaccines under development are HIV infections; acquired immunodeficiency syndrome (AIDS); pancreatic, breast, lung, colonic and prostatic cancers; multiple sclerosis; and stroke.

Nineteen biotechnology medicines are under development for auto-immune disorders, including 11 for rheumatoid arthritis and three for lupus; and eight for blood disorders, of which four are for haemophilia and one for sickle-cell disease.

The first medicine developed using biotechnology tools was a genetically engineered human insulin in 1982. Over the ensuing 16 years, 53 other biotechnology products were approved.

Equally importantly, the issuing of MAAs for these biotechnology products in the EU has been undertaken via a new centralised procedure, in which a company needs to obtain only a single marketing authorisation to be able to market the products throughout all 15 Member States. An explanation of the centralised procedure and the other avenues for obtaining a marketing authorisation is given in Chapter 2.

Preclinical pharmacotoxicological testing

Before any drug candidate is given to humans, extensive pharmacotoxicological testing in animals has to be undertaken to assess the potential for harmful as well as beneficial effects. There has been considerable debate both within and without the pharmaceutical industry about the use of animals in drug testing and the means by which their use can be minimised. The EU highlighted its commitment to reducing animal studies by establishing a European Centre for the Validation of Alternative Methods (ECVAM) in Ispra, Italy, in 1991 as part of the Environment Institute of the EU Joint Research Centre.

It is highly unlikely that it will be possible to replace all preclinical animal studies. However, ethical considerations require that their use should be minimised, and ways investigated in which such studies might be replaced by *in vitro* tests.[8] The criteria for reducing *in vivo* toxicology studies include avoiding replication of studies (e.g. between the USA, Europe and Japan); eliminating animal studies whose extrapolation to human studies has been found to be irrelevant; using new methodologies as they become available; and replacing *in vivo* tests, where possible, by human cell tests *in vitro*. Those *in vivo* toxicology studies which have already started to be replaced by *in vitro* tests include:

- assessment of toxicity by single-dose and repeated-dose administration
- evaluation of toxicity on reproductive function
- evaluation of carcinogenicity and mutagenicity.

Clinical studies

The assessment of the potential medicinal product in humans is the crux of the development of a new compound. If the product does not produce the expected effects in human studies, or produces unexpected and unwanted effects, the development programme for that compound will invariably fail at this stage. The potential for failure at this stage is high and, because of the already considerable financial investment in the compound, the later in the clinical studies that it occurs, the more severe the outcome is for the potential viability of the company. Moreover, knowledge of late clinical study failures often has a detrimental effect on the share price and market perception of the company concerned.

Phase I clinical studies

The initial studies in humans are carried out in 50–100 healthy volunteers (who do not have the condition under investigation, or any other illness) and conducted under the close supervision of a qualified medical doctor. Initial doses will be as low as possible to produce an expected effect; this will often be the same as the expected therapeutic dose, or the dose will be gradually increased to the expected therapeutic dose.

Up to May 2004, there was no requirement to obtain a clinical trial authorisation from the Medicines and Healthcare products Regulatory Agency (MHRA) before starting a Phase I trial. Approval to conduct the trial was required only from an ethics committee. However, under Directive 2001/20/EC on clinical trials, which was passed by the European Parliament in May 2001 and came into force in May 2004, studies carried out in healthy volunteers do require prior approval from the MHRA.

Despite the relatively small number of individuals involved, a well-conducted Phase I trial can accumulate much valuable information that is essential for the development programme to go forward to the next phase. Before any further studies can be undertaken, a further application for a clinical trial authorisation must be made to the MHRA for permission to carry out Phase II trials. (Prior to the new legislation being introduced, the MHRA had normally issued only a Clinical Trial Exemption (CTX) Certificate within 28 days of submission of the application, not a Clinical

Trial Certificate (CTC). Only for a limited number of 'problem' drugs was a full CTC required, and obtaining this was a considerably lengthier process. The scientific, medical and technical data requirements were the same for both a CTC and CTX. However, submission only of summaries of the data was required for a CTX application.)

Phase II clinical studies

These studies are the first time that the potential medicinal product has been given to patients (and frequently only to men if there is a lack of information on reproductive function) with the actual condition that the compound is intended to treat. In order to ascertain the correct dosage levels for therapeutic effects and unwanted side-effects, the drug is given to different groups of patients at different dosages. The number of patients treated in such trials is still relatively small, numbering between 200 and 400.

Phase III clinical studies

Again, after satisfactory completion of Phase II studies, the major clinical trials are initiated which will determine the fate of the drug. A local ethics committee must study the clinical trial protocol and approve the trial before it can start. In order to assess the effects statistically, more than 3000 patients are usually treated. Some patients are given the drug under test, some a placebo product (but identical in appearance). Alternatively, the drug may be tested against a known market leader, again with both products appearing identical. The doctors whose patients are enrolled in the studies are unaware whether their patients are receiving the test drug or the placebo/market leader. This is to prevent expectations from the doctor affecting the patient's perception (and reporting) of the effects generated by the product they are taking. The administered products are also usually switched during the trial, without the patients' or their prescriber's knowledge. These 'double-blind' trials have proved the most effective way to ensure objective and statistical assessment of the treatment under investigation.

Once the study is complete and the trials have been statistically analysed, the company can decide whether it wishes to collate the data to submit an MAA to a regulatory authority for the medicinal product. A listing of EU regulatory authorities is given in Appendix 1.

Post-marketing studies

It is only once a marketing authorisation has been given for the medicinal product that the product will be used in large populations of patients. As a result, and despite all the care that will have been exerted during clinical trials to ensure the product is safe and effective, it is only at this stage that unexpected problems with the product are likely to emerge. The drug is being used in an uncontrolled environment: there are no clinical trial associates to ensure that the doctor is prescribing the drug at the approved dosage; and doctors will be less intent on ensuring that patients are taking the medicinal product in the prescribed dosage.

Pharmacovigilance reports are requested from prescribers whose patients have experienced adverse effects from newly approved products. In the UK, the inverted black triangle (▼) is used by the UK regulatory authority, the MHRA, in the *British National Formulary*, and in other published prescribing sources to alert prescribers to newly approved products that require special attention to their use. Yellow report forms and prepaid yellow cards are available for doctors and hospital pharmacists to send to the MHRA in London and to Committee on Safety of Medicines (CSM) regional centres in Birmingham, Cardiff, Liverpool and Newcastle, reporting suspected adverse events. Community pharmacists have also been encouraged to submit suspected adverse reactions, following consultation by the pharmacist with the patient's doctor. However, the numbers of such reports from community pharmacists is disappointingly extremely small.[9]

If there are large numbers of these reports, the indications or dosage for the medicinal product may be restricted or, in severe cases, the product will be withdrawn from the market on instruction of the regulatory authority. In the EU, a withdrawal in one country automatically triggers assessment of the new medicinal product in the other Member States, and can lead to withdrawals being authorised throughout the Community.

References

1. Industrial Pharmacists Group. Salary survey 2000. *The Pharmaceutical Journal* 2000; **266**: 9.
2. The Impact of Economic and Political Factors on Pharmaceutical Innovation, Annual Centre for Medicines Research lecture, Raymond Gilmartin, CEO of Merck & Co. Quoted in *Health Horizons* 1998(Autumn); **35**: 13.
3. Hall M, Kirkness B (eds). *An A to Z of British Medicines Research*, 2nd edn. London: Association of the British Pharmaceutical Industry, 1998.
4. ABPI, *Pharmaceutical Facts and Statistics*, www.abpi.org.uk/statistics (accessed April 2003).
5. Source: Quoted in reference 4.
6. European Commission. *The Rules Governing Medicinal Products in the European Union.* Volume 1: *Pharmaceutical Legislation – medicinal products for human use.* Volume 2: *Notice to Applicants – medicinal products for human use.* Volume 3: *Guidelines – medicinal products for human use.* Volume 4: *Good Manufacturing Practices – medicinal products for human and veterinary use.* Volume 5: *Pharmaceutical Legislation – medicinal products for veterinary use.* Volume 6: *Notice to Applicants – medicinal products for veterinary use.* Volume 7: *Guidelines – medicinal products for veterinary*

use. Volume 8: *Maximum Residue Limits – veterinary medicinal products*. Volume 9: *Pharmacovigilance – medicinal products for human and veterinary use*. Luxembourg: European Commission, 1997–98.
7. PhRMA (Pharmaceutical Research and Manufacturers of America) survey, January 1999, www.phrma.org (accessed May 2003).
8. Committee for Proprietary Medicinal Products (CPMP) Position Paper CPMP/SWP/728/95, Replacement of animal studies by *in vitro* models, February 1995.
9. Harman RJ. The pivotal role of post-licensing activities, *BIRA Regulatory Review*, 1998; **1** (July): 3–8 and 1998; **1** (August): 6–10.

2

Options in the registration of medicinal products

Quality, safety and efficacy form the three principal criteria that must be satisfied by a company to market a medicinal product. These criteria form the basis of both the structure of the marketing authorisation application (MAA) and the registration process. Scientific assessment of medicinal product data is carried out by a regulatory authority, which may be national (e.g. the UK Medicines and Healthcare products Regulatory Agency, MHRA) or supranational (e.g. the European Agency for the Evaluation of Medicinal Products, EMEA). Details of regulatory authorities within the EU are given in Appendix 1, and the work undertaken by the MHRA for medicinal products is described in Chapter 9.

The MAA is divided into four elements:[1]

Part I A summary of the most important aspects of the application
Part II Data supporting the quality properties of the medicinal product
Part III Data supporting the pharmacotoxicological properties of the medicinal product
Part IV Data supporting the clinical properties of the medicinal product

Prior to the introduction of high-density computer storage media (e.g. CD-ROMs), the physical size of an MAA could be daunting. A paper-based application would invariably comprise hundreds of box files and ring files, with just its transfer to the regulatory authority demanding a major logistical exercise. Specially adapted software has assisted the production, management and cross-referencing within the MAA, but the correct and timely completion of such a vast undertaking is very expensive and complex – quite apart from the time and expense of the research needed to generate the product.

A further major consideration on the format and presentation of an MAA to any regulatory authority worldwide came into effect in 2003. The Common Technical Document (CTD) was created under the auspices of the ICH process (see Chapter 13), which has been an administrative process undertaken by the EU, the USA and Japan intended to harmonise the requirements for data submission. The CTD does not significantly alter the actual data required to support an MAA submitted in each of the three major regions of the world, but is intended to harmonise and standardise the way in which those data are presented. Doing so should reduce the amount of preparation time for the applicant and help harmonise the way in which the submitted data are assessed.

Part I: Summary of the dossier

As described in Chapter 1, Table 1.1, Part I of the EU MAA consists of the following:

Part IA   Administrative data
Part IB 1   Summary of Product Characteristics (SPC)
Part IB 2   Proposal for packaging, labelling and package insert
Part IB 3   SPCs already approved in the Member States
Part IC   Expert Reports on:
- chemical, pharmaceutical and biological documentation
- pharmacotoxicological (preclinical) documentation
- clinical documentation

Part IA: Administrative data

This Part is a summary of the content of the MAA, providing in effect a checklist that all required data have been submitted. It covers the following:

- the type of MAA (i.e. national, centralised, or one involving mutual recognition)
- the legal basis of the MAA (i.e. a full or abridged MAA, or a variation on an already approved MAA)
- the type of product covered by the MAA (i.e. a product containing a new active substance; a new strength or new pharmaceutical form of an already approved pharmaceutical; or a different route of administration of an already approved pharmaceutical)
- other countries in which the MAA has been approved or rejected.

Part IB 1: Summary of Product Characteristics (SPC)

It is the applicant company's responsibility to submit a draft SPC to the regulatory authority with the MAA. The SPC is one of the most important documents associated with the MAA. Its purpose and scope is set out in Directive 83/570/EEC, which states:

'It is necessary, from the point of view of public health and the free movement of medicinal products [within the EU], for the Competent Authorities to have at their disposal all useful information on authorised medicinal products, based in particular on summaries, adopted in other Member States, of the characteristics of products.'

The SPC encapsulates the findings of the assessment process, providing a statement of all aspects of the medicinal product agreed between the regulatory authority and the applicant company. When mutual recognition is initiated, the SPC produced by the initial assessing regulatory authority – termed the Reference Member State (RMS) (see page 21) – defines the nature and character of the medicinal product. It is impossible to amend the SPC without approval of the RMS.

In the UK, an annual publication of the Association of the British Pharmaceutical Industry (ABPI) and Datapharm Communications Ltd is the *Medicines Compendium,* available as both electronic and paper versions. This resource provides more than 2500 SPCs in a standardised format for prescribers and pharmacists. As prescribers are primarily interested in the clinical properties of the product, the section on 'Clinical particulars' precedes the sections on 'Pharmacological Properties' and 'Pharmaceutical Particulars' (in direct contradiction of the order of data submitted in an EU MAA). Table 2.1 outlines the agreed format of the SPC.

Part IC: Expert Reports

In Expert Reports, recognised experts on quality, safety and efficacy act as 'advocates' for the data contained in the MAA. The Expert Reports confirm that the requirements of appropriate guidelines have been followed; if the guidelines have not been followed, any deviations have to be justified.

Table 2.1 Summary of Product Characteristics – list of headings (Directive 83/570/EEC)

1. Trade name of the medicinal product
2. Qualitative and quantitative composition
3. Pharmaceutical form
4. Clinical particulars
    - 4.1 Therapeutic indications
    - 4.2 Posology and method of administration
    - 4.3 Contraindications
    - 4.4 Special warnings and special precautions for use
    - 4.5 Interaction with other medicaments and other forms of interaction
    - 4.6 Pregnancy and lactation
    - 4.7 Effects on ability to drive and use machines
    - 4.8 Undesirable effects
    - 4.9 Overdose
5. Pharmacological properties
    - 5.1 Pharmacodynamic properties
    - 5.2 Pharmacokinetic properties
    - 5.3 Preclinical safety data
6. Pharmaceutical particulars
    - 6.1 List of excipients
    - 6.2 Incompatibilities
    - 6.3 Shelf-life
    - 6.4 Special precautions for storage
    - 6.5 Nature and contents of container
    - 6.6 Instruction for use/handling
7. Marketing authorisation holder
8. Marketing authorisation number
9. Date of first authorisation/renewal of authorisation
10. Date of (partial) revision of the text

Guidance[2] has been issued on the format of Expert Reports. They should comprise a one- to two-page 'product profile', which in effect summarises the SPC, followed by a critical appraisal of the product's properties. Recommendations are given for the approximate lengths of the critical assessment part of each report:

- Quality: less than 10 pages
- Safety: less than 25 pages
- Efficacy: less than 25 pages.

Following the critical assessment portion of the Expert Report, the second part of the Expert Report comprises a tabular summary, giving a logical and concise presentation of the data. A tabular summary alone is deemed adequate for the quality Expert Report and the toxicological section of the safety Expert Report. Additional written summaries are recommended for the Expert Reports covering pharmacological safety issues (of not more than 10 pages) and efficacy issues (usually of a maximum of 30 pages). It should be understood that these documents comprise a very small part of the 200–300 volumes of data that a company has to assemble as a complete MAA.

Development of legislative controls for medicines

Early UK legislation

The Medicines Act was given Royal Assent in October 1968. It consolidated and expanded existing, but inadequate, legislation and became operative on 1 September 1971. The Act covered all aspects of the development, manufacture, packaging and labelling, distribution and advertising of medicinal products for human and veterinary use. It put on a statutory footing the activities of the former Committee on Safety of Drugs for human medicinal products.

The Medicines Act created the Medicines Commission, which advises the UK regulatory authority for human medicines, the Medicines and Healthcare products Regulatory Agency (MHRA), and ministers (the Licensing Authority) on matters relating to medicinal products. The Medicines Commission in turn advises on the setting up of specialist committees, which currently comprise:

- Advisory Board on the Registration of Homoeopathic Products
- British Pharmacopoeia Commission
- Committee on Safety of Medicines (CSM; which superseded the Committee on Safety of Drugs)
- Veterinary Products Committee.

The CSM has established three subcommittees to support its work:

- Chemistry, Pharmacy and Standards
- Biologicals
- Pharmacovigilance.

More recently, two further committees have been set up:

- Independent Review Panel for Advertising
- Independent Review Panel on the Classification of Borderline Substances.

The Medicines Commission and the above 'Section 4 Advisory Committees' (formed under Section 4 of the 1968 Medicines Act) must be consulted before a decision is taken by the Licensing Authority to refuse an MAA. They must also be consulted should it be necessary to revoke, vary or suspend a marketing authorisation on grounds of quality, safety and efficacy.

Initial Pan-European legislation

A legislative framework was developed in Europe at the same time as the introduction of the Medicines Act in the UK. European legislation has had an increasingly important influence on the control of medicines in the UK, especially since the early 1990s. The first legislation adopted by the then six members of the European Economic Community (EEC) was Directive 65/65/EEC; this still forms the basis for existing legislation. The UK joined the EEC in 1973, and the second phase of EEC legislation for pharmaceuticals was adopted in 1975.

The programme to create a single market in pharmaceuticals was begun by the implementation of Directive 75/319/EEC. This established a Committee for Proprietary Medicinal Products (CPMP) to help Member States agree to decisions relating to the control of medicines. A new 'multistate' procedure (initially called the CPMP procedure) to assess and approve marketing authorisations was also established. This was intended to minimise duplication of the assessment procedures for MAAs in different countries and to promote a harmonised market for pharmaceuticals throughout Europe. However, there was a marked reluctance by Member States to agree to the assessments carried out by other regulatory authorities and almost all MAAs had to be referred to the CPMP for arbitration.

At the same time as the introduction of the multistate procedure, Directive 75/320/EEC established a Pharmaceutical Committee. This had members from all Member States and was formed to advise the European Commission on policy matters relating to medicinal products.

In 1987 a further authorisation procedure, the concertation procedure, was introduced by Directive 87/22/EEC. Its use was mandatory for biotechnology products and optional for high-technology products. Member States could consult each other when carrying out the assessment of these complex medicines, and the new system proved moderately successful.

At the same time as implementing changes to the major legislation affecting MAAs, the European Community (EC) (as it had by then become) generated many other Directives that affected all Member States, including the UK. These covered all aspects of the marketing of medicinal products for human use.

Existing UK and European legislation

It was realised that neither the multistate nor concertation procedures had proved as successful as had been hoped. Consequently, a major review of approval procedures was begun in the late 1980s, culminating in what was then called the 'Future Systems' package. This comprised:

- EC Regulation No. 2309/93, which established a new European regulatory authority, the EMEA, and a new centralised procedure for obtaining a marketing authorisation (see below)
- Directive 93/39/EEC for human medicinal products, which amended Directives 65/65/EEC, 75/318/EEC, and 75/319/EEC
- Directive 93/41/EEC which repealed Directive 87/22/EEC.

The launch date for the 'Future Systems' legislative package was 1 January 1995. The legislation is the basis of the current system of approval of medicinal products in the UK and the rest of the (now renamed) European Union (EU). Under the legislation, MAAs for medicinal products can be authorised by one of two means.

The centralised procedure

The passage of European Council Regulation (EC) No. 2309/93 created for the first time a means by which companies could obtain a single marketing authorisation for a medicinal product that is valid across the entire EU. Co-ordination of the assessment of centralised MAAs is the responsibility of the EMEA. The scientific assessment of a centralised MAA is carried out by the Committee for Proprietary Medicinal Products (CPMP) (for human medicinal products) and by the Committee for Veterinary Medicinal Products (CVMP) (for veterinary medicinal products). The CPMP/CVMP appoints one of its members to act as the co-ordinator and primary assessor (rapporteur) for the passage of the MAA through the centralised route. Companies can suggest up to three or four Committee members whom it would like to act as rapporteur, and the EMEA tries to satisfy the company's choice(s).

Use of the centralised route is mandatory for medicinal products derived from biotechnology. Such products are described as Part A products. It is possible that its use may become mandatory for all new chemical entities under the ongoing review of legislation (see page 27).

Companies have the option of using the centralised procedure for MAAs for products that are deemed 'innovative', with novel characteristics. Such products are referred to as Part B products. The definition of 'innovative' includes:

- a new delivery system
- an entirely new indication for an already approved medicinal product
- where the medicinal product's action is based on the presence of radioisotopes; and
- entirely new active substances.

Examples of products that were approved via the centralised procedure during 1998[3] are given in Table 2.2.

The mutual recognition procedure

The mutual recognition procedure is controlled by Directives 93/39/EEC (for human medicines) and 93/40/EEC (for veterinary medicines) and by Regulation No. 541/95 (used for varying the terms of marketing authorisations). Under the mutual recognition procedure, one of the EU national regulatory authorities (the RMS) undertakes the assessment of the MAA against the scientific criteria of quality, safety and efficacy. If approved, a national marketing authorisation is issued. The details of the authorisation are then sent to other 'Concerned Member States' in which the pharmaceutical company wishes to market the product. These Concerned Member States are intended to mutually recognise the authorisation.

The MAA's assessment by this first Member State must be completed within 210 days of submission. Subsequently, the applicant company can ask the initial Member State in which the assessment was carried out – the RMS – to obtain approval of the authorisation in one or more other EU Member States. Assessment by further Member States must be completed within 90 days. Other Member States can object to the approval by the RMS only if they have serious grounds for believing the product to be a risk to public health within their territories.

Table 2.2 A selection of products that were approved via the EU centralised procedure in 1998

Drug name	Proprietary name	Manufacturer(s)	Indications
Pramipexole	Mirapexin	Pharmacia and Upjohn SV	Parkinson's disease
Interferon beta-1a	Rebif	Serono	Multiple sclerosis
Clopidogrel	Iscover	Bristol-Myers Squib	Prevention of vascular ischaemia
Sildenafil	Viagra	Pfizer Limited UK	Erectile dysfunction
Telmisartan	Telmisartan	Boehringer Ingelheim	Hypertension
Rivastigmine	Prometax	Novartis Europharm	Alzheimer's disease
Emedastine	Emadine	Alcon Laboratories (UK)	Allergic conjunctivitis

A key requirement for mutual recognition is that the MAA submitted to Concerned Member States is identical in all respects to that approved by the RMS. If mutual recognition is requested early in the life of the medicinal product, this is usually not a problem. If a mutual recognition request has been deferred for any reason, it may be necessary to update the original MAA dossier and the Expert Reports in the light of later scientific knowledge or clinical experience with the product. This must be done with the full agreement and knowledge of the RMS.

Mutual recognition is open to all classes of medicinal products except two: it cannot be applied to a product authorised under the centralised procedure (see details above) or to homoeopathic medicinal products.

Application of the 'Future Systems' legislation in the UK

The UK Medicines Act was not deemed suitable for transposing many of the new European Directives (the EU Regulation was automatically effective in all Member States). As a result, new UK legislation was promulgated, called The Medicines for Human Use (Marketing Authorisations Etc.) Regulations 1994, which became effective on 1 January 1995. The UK Regulations provided legislation that cross-referred to the European legislation rather than setting out the texts in full. This method of implementation was chosen to minimise the duplication of UK and EU law, to ensure that the EU law was implemented in full, and to minimise potential complications when later changes were made to EU legislation.

In essence, the UK Medicines for Human Use (Marketing Authorisations Etc.) Regulations 1994 provide the following controls:

- the requirements for MAAs and the procedures for granting, varying and renewing marketing authorisations
- obligations imposed upon UK marketing authorisation holders, including pharmacovigilance requirements
- labelling and package leaflet requirements
- provisions relating to the Licensing Authority to suspend, compulsorily vary or revoke a marketing authorisation
- related enforcement measures.

Framework legislation for pharmaceuticals

The most important legislation that has been introduced in the EU, and which has direct relevance to UK legislation, is listed in Table 2.3.

Provision of advice to applicant companies

The criteria to achieve a successful marketing authorisation are the same in both the centralised and mutual recognition procedures (see above). Similarly, companies may seek scientific advice to assist them in the product development process: from the RMS for a submission through the mutual

Table 2.3 Important legislation for medicinal products for human use in Europe

Reference number	Title
Directives	
65/65/EEC	On the approximation of provisions laid down by law, regulation or administrative action relating to medicinal products
75/318/EEC	On the approximation of the laws of Member States relating to the analytical, pharmacotoxicological and clinical standards and protocols in respect of testing of medicinal products
75/319/EEC	On the approximation of provisions laid down by law, regulation or administrative action relating to medicinal products
89/105/EEC	Relating to the transparency of measures regulating the pricing of medicinal products for human use and their inclusion within the scope of national health insurance schemes
89/342/EEC	Extending the scope of Directives 65/65/EEC and 75/319/EEC and laying down additional provisions for immunological medicinal products consisting of vaccines, toxins, or serums and allergens
89/343/EEC	Extending the scope of Directives 65/65/EEC and 75/319/EEC and laying down additional provisions for radiopharmaceuticals
89/381/EEC	Extending the scope of Directives 65/65/EEC and 75/319/EEC and laying down additional provision on the approximation of provisions laid down by law, regulation or administrative action relating to proprietary medicinal products and laying down special provisions for medicinal products derived from human blood or human plasma
91/356/EEC	Laying down the principles and guidelines of good manufacturing practice for medicinal products for human use
92/25/EEC	On the wholesale distribution of medicinal products for human use
92/26/EEC	Concerning the classification for the supply of medicinal products for human use
92/27/EEC	On the labelling of medicinal products for human use and on package leaflets
92/28/EEC	On the advertising of medicinal products for human use
92/73/EEC	Widening the scope of Directives 65/65/EEC and 75/319/EEC on the approximation of provisions laid down by law, regulation or administrative action relating to medicinal products and laying down additional provisions on homoeopathic medicinal products
93/39/EEC	Amending Directives 65/65/EEC, 75/318/EEC, and 75/319/EEC in respect of medicinal products
93/41/EEC	Repealing Directive 87/22/EEC on the approximation of national measures relating to the placing of high-technology medicinal products, especially those derived from biotechnology
2001/20/EC	Relating to the implementation of good clinical practice in the conduct of clinical trials on medicinal products for human use
2001/83/EC	On the Community Code relating to medicinal products for human use

continued

Table 2.3 Important legislation for medicinal products for human use in Europe (*cont.*)

Reference number	Title
Regulations	
EEC 2309/93	Laying down Community procedures for the authorisation and supervision of medicinal products for human and veterinary use and establishing a European Agency for the Evaluation of Medicinal Products
EC 297/95	On fees payable to the European Agency for the Evaluation of Medicinal Products
EC 540/95	Laying down the arrangements for reporting suspected unexpected adverse reactions which are not serious, whether arising in the Community or a third country, to medicinal products for human or veterinary use authorised in accordance with the provisions of Council Regulation (EEC) No. 2309/93
EC 541/95	Concerning the examination of variations to the terms of a marketing authorisation granted by a competent authority of a Member State
EC 542/95	Concerning the examination of variations to the terms of a marketing authorisation falling within the scope of Council Regulation (EEC) No. 2309/93
EC 1662/95	Laying down certain detailed arrangements for implementing the Community decision-making procedures in respects of marketing authorisations for products for human or veterinary use

recognition procedure; and for centralised MAAs from the EMEA. Advice will usually only be given on topics that are currently not the subject of guidelines from the CPMP/CVMP or the European Commission. A request for advice must be made in writing, and the EMEA Secretariat or CPMP will determine whether the request warrants giving advice. CPMP advice may be given in writing or orally at meetings organised with the potential applicant company. While the CPMP is keen to assist applicants to the greatest extent possible, the advice given to the potential applicant company is not binding.

The importance attached by the EMEA to ensure that applicants receive maximum assistance is reflected by an opportunity to meet the EMEA Secretariat in a pre-MAA-submission meeting. Indeed, it has been shown that the passage of the MAA through the centralised procedure is facilitated by companies seeking advice from the EMEA 6 months before submission. The information that the EMEA might request at this time can include: a draft SPC; the justification for the company using the centralised procedure for its product; the company's preference for a rapporteur for its MAA, ideally suggesting three or four CPMP members from three or four different Member States (members sit on the CPMP for their personal scientific and medical expertise; they are not deemed to represent their national authority in their CPMP activities); and any regulatory issues or difficulties which might render the application nonstandard.

The submission timetable

On receipt of a centralised MAA, the dossier is evaluated by the Secretariat within 10 working days. The CPMP rapporteur coordinates the passage of the MAA through the centralised procedure. The MAA submitted as a centralised application should comprise one complete copy plus two additional copies of Part I of the data. The Part I data will include copies of the company's draft SPC, labelling and package leaflet in all 20 official EU languages of all Member States.

Subsequently, pre-authorisation inspections of manufacturing sites are co-ordinated by the EMEA. When these are completed, scientific evaluation can commence. As with MAAs submitted through the mutual recognition procedure, a centralised MAA must be assessed and an opinion given by the CPMP within 210 days of its validation. When the assessment is completed, CPMP issues an Opinion on the MAA which has been reached by scientific consensus. If scientific consensus cannot be achieved, then a majority Opinion will be produced. If the Opinion is favourable, the following documents are appended to it: a draft SPC; the conditions (if any) attached to an authorisation; a draft labelling and package leaflet; a legal classification under which the medicinal product can be supplied; and the Assessment Report, produced by the CPMP.

The applicant company has to produce relevant translations of these documents within 5 days of the CPMP Opinion. Over the subsequent 15 days, any comments made by CPMP members regarding these translations must be incorporated. Final translations are sent to the EMEA 20 days after the Opinion has been issued.

To ensure that the translations are valid, assessment of their quality is carried out by the EMEA in co-operation with Member States.

Issuing the marketing authorisation

The EMEA is not empowered to issue a marketing authorisation. For centralised applications, this must be done by the European Commission. The EMEA has 30 days to transmit to the Commission the Opinion and/or its Appendices. The Commission prepares a draft Decision on the proposed marketing authorisation by consultation with all members of the Commission. Following this, the draft decision is sent to the Pharmaceutical Standing Committee within a further 30 days. If the Standing Committee raises no objections, again within 30 days, the Decision is returned to the Commission and the Commission issues its final Decision.

In theory, the documentation on the medicinal product authorised during the centralised procedure should be identical in all Member States. However, the product label may be required in the language of the Member State; and certain Member States require additional labelling (e.g. the price of the medicinal product, the reimbursement conditions, and the legal status, plus the identification and authenticity of the marketing authorisation). What is consistent throughout all Member States is the marketing authorisation number, which must appear on the packaging. The Commission recognises the difficulties of having the year incorporated into the authorisation number, but issued guidance in September 1997 that a two-digit number '00' would be appropriate for products given a marketing authorisation in the year 2000. Once the final Decision has been reached and published, the marketing authorisation is granted for a period of 5 years and can be renewed if an application is made at least 3 months prior to expiry of the authorisation.

The Common Technical Document

The Common Technical Document (CTD) was developed as part of the process that has been ongoing since 1990 to harmonise the technical requirements for the registration of medicinal products for human use in the EU, the USA and Japan – the ICH process. (More information on the ICH process can be found in Chapter 13.)

Under the CTD format, the data in support of an MAA are divided into five modules:

Module 1:   Administrative and prescribing information (region specific)
Module 2:   Summaries and overview
Module 3:   Information on product quality
Module 4:   Nonclinical study reports
Module 5:   Clinical study reports.

Administrative and prescribing information (Module 1)

This is the one part of the MAA that has to be tailored to meet the specific requirements of the authority under whose remit the application is being submitted, and in effect is not part of the CTD.

All regions require a Table of Contents, which includes a summary of the information included in Module 1. All administrative documents (which include application forms, certificates and prescribing information) should also be provided. In essence, however, authorities can set their own requirements as to the information that is required in Module 1.

Summaries and overview (Module 2)

Following an overall CTD Table of Contents of Modules 2 to 5 inclusive, this part of the application should begin with a one-page summary of the medicinal product, which includes its therapeutic class, mode of action and proposed clinical use. Overviews and summaries of each of the succeeding sections of the MAA are to be provided as follows:

- quality overall summary
- nonclinical overview

- clinical overview
- nonclinical summary and tabulated summaries
- clinical summary.

The nonclinical summary and clinical summary documents should be provided in separate volumes to facilitate review.

Quality (Module 3), Nonclinical (Module 4) and Clinical (Module 5)

The information in each of these modules has a common format:

- Table of Contents
- body of data
- literature references.

Detailed guidance is given on the format, ordering and numbering of each of the sections within these modules. The use of standard presentation tools (e.g. tab dividers and binding dividers) is also recommended.

General issues

The CTD also gives guidance on the organisation of the information submitted. It covers the format of amendments and supplements, the binding of documents, and the number of copies required of each section of the submission. Paper size and margins are also specified, bearing in mind that paper sizes are different in different parts of the world. The colour of binder covers, the thickness of each volume, and their numbering and identification are also specified.

Guidance has also been issued on the format and style of an electronic CTD (eCTD) for submission in each of the three geographical regions.

Review of pharmaceutical legislation

Table 2.3 shows that a great number of Directives and Regulations have been introduced and implemented over a number of years into which, inevitably, inconsistencies were introduced. To overcome this, the legislation was recast into a single legislative text, Directive 2001/83/EC for human medicinal products, which is termed the Community Code and which supersedes all the previous texts.

In 1995, it had been agreed that a review of the new systems would take place after 5 years in operation, and the review of pharmaceutical legislation was started in 2000. The proposed changes are a consequence of the enlargement of the EU in 2004/5 to 25 Member States and of the experience gained by using the systems as they were implemented.

Proposed changes to the EMEA

The structure of the Agency and its Committees is to be changed. The CPMP is to be renamed the Committee for Human Medicinal Products (CHMP); representation from each Member State on the Committees is to be reduced; and the Agency's Management Board is to be restructured. A new Committee of Herbal Medicinal Products is to be formed to work alongside the CHMP, the Committee for Veterinary Medicinal Products (CVMP), and the Committee for Orphan Medicinal Products (COMP).

Proposed changes to the centralised procedure

It has been proposed to broaden the scope of the procedure so that it is mandatory for all new medicinal products for human use containing a new active substance for which the therapeutic indication is the treatment of AIDS, cancer, neurodegenerative disorders or diabetes. Other proposals are to shorten the time allowed for assessment of applications, introduce fast-track procedures for major innovative products, remove the 5-year expiry date for authorisations, and increase the number of safety reports that the company holding the authorisation has to produce.

Proposed changes to the mutual recognition procedure

The timescale for carrying out the assessment of an application is to be reduced from 210 days to 150 days, and the legislative framework for post-marketing pharmacovigilance is to be strengthened so that urgent action by one Member State must be implemented at a Community level.

References

1. European Commission. *The Rules Governing Medicinal Products in the European Union*, Vol. 2A, *Notice to Applicants: medicinal products for human use; procedures for marketing authorisation*. Luxembourg: European Commission, 1998.
2. The European Agency for the Evaluation of Medicinal Products (EMEA), *4th General Report 1998*, December 1998, London: EMEA.
3. For products approved under the centralised procedure: Commission Regulation No. 542/95 of 10 March 1995 concerning the examination of variations to the terms of a marketing authorisation falling within the scope of Council Regulation (EEC) No. 2309/93. *Official Journal of the European Communities* 1995; L55: 15.

3

Quality issues

Quality issues cover all aspects of the chemical, pharmaceutical and biological development of a new product. They are covered in Part II of the marketing authorisation application (MAA).[1] In essence, this covers the following for ingredients and finished products:

- their composition
- method of preparation
- the control of starting materials
- control tests carried out on intermediate products
- control tests on the finished product
- stability data
- bioavailablility and bioequivalence *in vitro*
- data related to the environment risk assessment of products containing genetically modified organisms (GMOs)
- other information.

Coverage of these elements of pharmaceutical development is essential for all products for human or veterinary use: chemically active substances, radiopharmaceutical products, biological medicinal products, or vegetable medicinal products. Some variation does occur, however, in the requirements for specific members of these groups.

In order to assist applicants in the EU provide the necessary information for each of the above topics, guidelines or Notes for Guidance have been produced by the EU Committee for Proprietary Medicinal Products (CPMP) (sometimes in conjunction with the Committee for Veterinary Medicinal Products (CVMP)) of the European Agency for the Evaluation of Medicinal Products (EMEA). Although these have no legislative standing, applicants must justify their own processes where they differ from those given in the published guidelines. Adopted and draft EU 'quality' guidelines are listed in Table 3.1. Those that are currently under development within the International Conference on Harmonisation of the Technical Requirements for the Registration of Pharmaceuticals for Human Use (ICH) and which are therefore also to be adopted within the EU, are listed in Table 3.2.

The CPMP Quality Working Group has also produced Concept Papers that discuss at greater length than the Notes for Guidance particular important issues. Those currently available are listed in Table 3.3.

The guidelines on quality aspects of the MAA are published as a compendium in Volume 3A of *The Rules Governing Medicinal Products in*

Table 3.1 Adopted and draft quality guidelines

Guidelines adopted by the joint Quality Working Party (QWP) of the Committee for Proprietary Medicinal Products (CPMP) (and some in conjunction with the Committee for Veterinary Medicinal Products (CVMP)) of the European Agency for the Evaluation of Medicinal Products (EMEA). Copyright EMEA. Situation as at December 2003

Reference number	Title
Adopted guidelines	
CPMP/QWP/158/01 Revision (CVMP/115/01)	Note for Guidance on Quality of water for pharmaceutical use (Revision adopted by CPMP/CVMP May 02)
CPMP/QWP/2845/00	Note for Guidance on Requirements for pharmaceutical documentation for pressurised metered dose inhalation products (CPMP adopted Mar. 02)
CPMP/QWP/1719/00	Note for Guidance on Medicinal gases: pharmaceutical documentation (CPMP adopted Jan. 02)
CPMP/QWP/2820/00 (EMEA/CVMP/815/00)	Note for Guidance on Specifications: test procedures and acceptance criteria for herbal drugs, herbal drug preparations and herbal medicinal products (CPMP/CVMP adopted July 01)
CPMP/QWP/2819/00 (EMEA/CVMP/814/00)	Note for Guidance on Quality of herbal medicinal products (CPMP/CVMP adopted July 01)
CPMP/QWP/072/96	CPMP/CVMP Note for Guidance on Start of shelf-life of the finished dosage form (Annex to the Note for Guidance on the Manufacture of the finished dosage form) (Adopted by CPMP/CVMP May 2001)
CPMP/QWP/159/01 (CVMP/271/01)	Note for Guidance on Limitations to the use of ethylene oxide in the manufacture of medicinal products (CPMP/CVMP adopted Mar. 01)
CPMP/QWP/848/96 (EMEA/CVMP/598/99)	Note for Guidance on Process validation (CPMP/CVMP adopted Feb. 01)
CPMP/QWP/3015/99	Note for Guidance on Parametric release (CPMP adopted Feb. 01)
CPMP/QWP/2934/99	Note for Guidance for In-use stability testing of human medicinal products – Annex to Note for Guidance on Stability testing of existing active substances and related finished products and Note for Guidance on Stability testing of new drug substances and products (CPMP adopted Feb. 01)
CPMP/QWP/604/96	Note for Guidance on Quality of modified release products: a. oral dosage forms; b. and transdermal dosage forms; Section I (quality)
CPMP/QWP/8567/99	Explanatory note on the operation of two-year transition period for application of Note for Guidance on residual solvents to marketed products
CPMP/QWP/054/98	Annex to Note for Guidance on Development pharmaceutics (CPMP/QWP/155/96): Decision trees for selection of sterilisation methods
CPMP/CVMP/QWP/115/95	Note for Guidance on Inclusion of antioxidants and antimicrobial preservatives in medicinal products

continued

Table 3.1 Adopted and draft quality guidelines (*cont.*)

Reference number	Title
CPMP/QWP/158/96	Note for Guidance on Dry powder inhalers
CPMP/QWP/576/96	Note for Guidance on Stability testing for a Type II variation to a marketing authorisation (CPMP adopted Apr. 98)
CPMP/QWP/556/96	Note for Guidance on Stability testing of existing active substances and related finished products (CPMP adopted Apr. 98)
CPMP/QWP/297/97	Note for Guidance on Summary of requirements for active substances in Part II of the dossier (CPMP adopted Jan. 98)
CPMP/QWP/155/96	Note for Guidance on Development pharmaceutics (CPMP adopted Jan. 98)
CPMP/QWP/609/96	Note for Guidance on Declaration of storage conditions for medicinal products particulars and active substances (Annex to Note for Guidance on Stability testing of new active substances and medicinal products, Annex to Note for Guidance on Stability of existing active substances and related finished products) (CPMP adopted Jan. 98)
CPMP/QWP/159/96	Note for Guidance on Maximum shelf-life for sterile products after first opening or following reconstitution (CPMP adopted Jan. 98)
CPMP/QWP/486/95	Note for Guidance on Manufacture of the finished dosage form (CPMP adopted Sept. 95)
Draft guidelines	
CPMP/QWP/122/02	Note for Guidance on Stability testing of existing active substances and related finished products (Released for consultation, Feb. 02)
CPMP/QWP/227/02 (EMEA/CVMP/134/02)	Note for Guidance on the European Drug Master File procedure (Released for consultation, Feb. 02)
CPMP/QWP/609/96 Rev. 1	Note for Guidance on Declaration of storage conditions for medicinal products particulars and active substances (Annex to Note for Guidance on Stability testing of new active substances and medicinal products, Annex to Note for Guidance on Stability of existing active substances and related finished products) (Released for consultation, Dec. 01)
CPMP/QWP/130/96 Rev. 1	Note for Guidance on Chemistry of the new active substance (Re-released for consultation, Dec. 01)
CPMP/QWP/3309/01 (EMEA/CVMP/961/01)	Note for Guidance on the Use of near infrared spectroscopy by the pharmaceutical industry and the data to be forwarded in the Part II of the dossier for a marketing authorisation (Re-released for consultation, Nov. 01)
CPMP/EWP/QWP/1401/98	Note for Guidance on the Investigation of bioavailability and bioequivalence (Re-released for consultation, Dec. 2000)

Table 3.2 ICH adopted and draft quality guidelines

Guidelines which have been developed or which are under development under the auspices of the International Conference on the Harmonisation of the Technical Requirements for the Registration of Pharmaeuticals for Human Use (ICH). Situation as at December 2003

Reference number	Title
Adopted guidelines	
CPMP/ICH/1940/00 – CPMP adopted 02	Note for Guidance on Impurities: residual solvents – permissible daily exposure (TDE) for tetrahydrofuran and N-methylpyrrolidone
CPMP/ICH/283/95 adopted Apr. 02	Maintenance for Note for Guidance on Impurities: residual solvents – type of maintenance: updating based on new information
CPMP/ICH/2737/99 (Revision of CPMP/ICH/142/95) – adopted Feb. 02	Note for Guidance on Impurities testing: impurities in new drug substances
CPMP/ICH/4104/00 – adopted Feb. 02	Note for Guidance on Bracketing and matrixing designs for stability testing of drug substances and drug products
CPMP/ICH/4106/00 – released for consultation July 2000	Note for Guidance on Good Manufacturing Practice for active pharmaceutical ingredients
CPMP/ICH/2736/99 (Revision of CPMP/ICH/380/95) – adopted Nov. 2000	Note for Guidance on Stability testing of new drug substances and products
CPMP/ICH/367/96 – adopted Nov. 99	Note for Guidance on Specifications: test procedures and acceptance criteria for new drug substances and new drug products: chemical substances
CPMP/ICH/365/96 – adopted Mar. 99	Note for Guidance on Specifications: test procedures and acceptance criteria for biotechnological/biological products
CPMP/ICH/283/95 – adopted Sept. 97	Note for Guidance on Impurities: residual solvents
CPMP/ICH/294/95 – adopted Sept. 97	Note for Guidance on Quality of biotechnological products: derivation and characterisation of cell substrates used for production of biotechnological/biological products
CPMP/ICH/295/95 – adopted Apr. 97	Note for Guidance on Quality of biotechnological products: viral safety evaluation of biotechnology products derived from cell lines of human or animal origin
CPMP/ICH/279/95 – adopted Dec. 96	Note for Guidance on Photostability testing of new active substances and medicinal products
CPMP/ICH/280/95 – adopted Dec. 96	Note for Guidance on Stability testing: requirements for new dosage forms
CPMP/ICH/281/95 – adopted Dec. 96	Note for Guidance on Validation of analytical procedures: methodology
CPMP/ICH/282/95 – adopted Dec. 96	Note for Guidance on Impurities in new medicinal products

continued

Table 3.2 ICH adopted and draft quality guidelines (*cont.*)

Reference number	Title
CPMP/ICH/142/95 – adopted May 95	Note for Guidance on Impurities testing: impurities in new drug substances
CPMP/ICH/380/95 – adopted Dec. 93	Note for Guidance on Stability testing: stability testing of new drug substances and products
CPMP/ICH/381/95 – adopted Nov. 94	Note for Guidance on Validation of analytical methods: definitions and terminology
CPMP/ICH/138/95 – adopted Dec. 95	Note for Guidance on Quality of biotechnological products: stability testing of biotechnological/biological products
CPMP/ICH/139/95 – adopted Dec. 95	Note for Guidance on Quality of biotechnological products: analysis of the expression construct in cell lines used for production of r-DNA derived protein products
Draft guidelines	
CPMP/ICH/420/02 – released for consultation Feb. 02	Note for Guidance on Evaluation of stability data
CPMP/ICH/421/02 – released for consultation Feb. 02	Note for Guidance on Stability data package for registration in climatic zones III and IV
CPMP/ICH/2738/99 (revision of CPMP/ICH/282/95) – released for consultation Nov. 99	Note for Guidance on Impurities in new drug products

Table 3.3 Quality Concept Papers

Concept Papers issued by the Quality Working Party (QWP) of the Committee for Proprietary Medicinal Products (CPMP) of the European Agency for the Evaluation of Medicinal Products (EMEA). Copyright EMEA. Situation as at December 2003

Reference number	Title
Concept papers	
CPMP/QWP/2930/99	Development of a CPMP Note for Guidance on Requirements for pharmaceutical documentation for metered dose inhalers
CPMP/QWP/2809/98 (corrected)	Revision of the Note for Guidance on Radiopharmaceuticals
CPMP/QWP/2430/98	Revision of the Note for Guidance on the European Drug Master File procedure for active substances
CPMP/QWP/2431/98	Development of a CPMP Note for Guidance on Parametric release
CPMP/QWP/2570/98	Development of a CPMP Note for Guidance on In-use stability testing of nonsterile human medicinal products

the European Union.[1] The following summary of quality requirements is based upon the guidelines published in this volume. (The numbering of EU guidelines is convoluted and inconsistent. Later documents, or earlier ones that have been the subject of revision, are numbered as in Tables 3.1 and 3.2; earlier ones still can only be referenced by their original EC designation. The designation in Volume 3A of the *Rules* is given in the discussion below.)

Development pharmaceutics and process validation (Note for Guidance III/847/87)

This guideline reflects the need for pharmaceutical development studies to be carried out to ensure that the dosage form and formulation of a proposed medicinal product are appropriate. Batch reproducibility is also critically ensured by compliance with the guideline.

Development pharmaceutics – constituents

These comprise the active substances and excipients. The active substance must be shown to be compatible with the excipients, and the effect of any variation in physical characteristics (e.g. particle size) on the formulation must be studied. If there is a risk that any change in physical characteristics may produce changes in bioavailability or any other actions of the formulation, the controls put in place to monitor this must be described. The presence of any overage produced during manufacturing must be justified.

The role of all excipients must be explained. If an unusual excipient is used, in order to produce a particular effect in the formulation, full information on the excipient must be given.

Composition

The requirements vary according to the type of dosage form. For liquid dosage forms, the effect of changes in physical characteristics must be demonstrated. The effect of changes in pH on the active ingredient must be shown. Other factors (e.g. ease of dissolution, and changes in aggregation) must also be considered. The inclusion of other nonexcipient additives (e.g. preservatives and antioxidants) must also be justified. If a product is to be given intravenously, compatibility with other products is of particular importance. For semi-solid dosage forms, similar considerations regarding pH and additives must be addressed.

Different issues affect solid dosage forms. Dissolution of a solid dosage form is critical, and the tests should be carried out for both non-modified-release and modified-release (e.g. prolonged-release) formulations. Correlation of *in vitro* with *in vivo* studies may be required for certain formulations.

It is essential that the mixture of active ingredient and excipients in a solid dosage form is uniform. Although the *European Pharmacopoeia* (PhEur) refers to single-dosage forms containing 2 mg per dose or less, the guideline states that homogeneity must be ensured for all solid dosage forms.

Container and closure

Any possible interaction between the container and closure and the formulated product must be documented. This can include the extraction from solution of one or more of the ingredients, which is especially problematic with glass and rubber container and closure materials. Possible leaching of ingredients must also be considered. If a dosing device is to be used, evidence must be presented that the dose received by the patient is reproducible.

Process validation

The concept of process validation deals with the manufacturing process and its quality. It is associated with Good Manufacturing Practice (GMP). It is, however, more concerned with nonstandard methods of manufacturing that might be used in the production process, and ensuring that they produce a final product of expected quality.

Manufacture of the finished dosage form (Note for Guidance III/3421/93)

This guideline covers:

- the MAA and GMP
- manufacturing formula
- description of the manufacturing process
- description of the manufacturing chain
- validation of the manufacturing process
- special items.

GMP is defined in EC Directive 91/356/EEC, and all medicinal products must be manufactured according to GMP. The MAA should contain information specific to the medicinal product under review, and general aspects of GMP need not be described. This guideline describes those elements of GMP that should be described.

Manufacturing formula

The product must be manufactured to a predefined formula. This includes information about the batch size, and any variations which might be allowed in the finished product batch size; the basic ingredients of the product, including their specifications and any overages which are allowed; and the variation in quantity (if any) which the formula permits in the use of individual ingredients (these must be specified for both the active ingredient(s) and excipients).

Description of the manufacturing process

This must be given, together with any variations in the manufacturing process which might be allowed in exceptional circumstances. The description should include the equipment used and the in-process controls which have been built into the manufacturing process. A flow-chart of the process is essential, although the level of detail should not be so specific as to be restrictive upon the manufacturer in making minor alterations. No major changes to the manufacturing process can be permitted unless previously agreed with the regulatory authority that issues the marketing authorisation. What is important is that the process produces a medicinal product of expected and known specification.

Description of the manufacturing chain

All sites where manufacturing and assembly of the product take place must be notified, even if the different sites belong to the same company. The name of the company responsible for final batch release must also be given.

Validation data of the manufacturing process

Process validation must be described if there are any doubts about the ability of the manufacturing process to guarantee the specifications of the finished product.

Special items

A range of 'special items' are included in the guideline to cover unusual manufacturing issues that might arise. These include any method of sterilisation used; the re-processing of any leftover manufactured product; the removal of solvents or gases; the cleaning and sterilisation of primary packaging material; and details of production areas.

Limitations to the use of ethylene oxide in the manufacture of medicinal products (Note for Guidance III/9261/90)

Toxicological background

The high potential carcinogenic effect of ethylene oxide has led to the recommendation in this guideline that the compound be used only when it is pharmaceutically essential to do so, and only when a limit of 1 part per million (ppm) is applied.

Categories of the use of ethylene oxide

The compound is a surface-only sterilising agent. Although it can be used on pharmaceutical raw materials, finished products and containers, its use on each occasion must be justified.

Specifications and test procedures

This covers the use of ethylene oxide on raw materials, the finished product and containers.

The use of ionising radiation in the manufacture of medicinal products (Note for Guidance III/9109/90)

The need for microbial decontamination and sterilisation (e.g. of starting materials, packaging materials and finished products) in the manufacture of medicinal products may require the use of ionising radiation. Additional information to that given in this guideline on the use of ionising radiation is found in an Annex within Volume 4 of *The Rules Governing Medicinal Products in the European Union*.[2]

Administrative data

Full details of the product to be irradiated are required and the stage of the manufacturing process the material is at (e.g. whether it is a starting material or a finished product). Batch size data are also required. The purpose of the irradiation must be given, with the minimum dose to achieve this and the maximum permissible dose that can be used. The manufacturer's details must also be given and the location of the sites where irradiation is carried out.

Manufacturing process

Descriptions of the irradiation plant and process must be given. Full details of the passage of the product through the irradiation process are required (e.g. the dimensions and material of the irradiation container, and the loading pattern of the container within the irradiation unit).

Validation of the irradiation procedure

Validation details must relate to the procedure and dose, the purpose of the irradiation, and the quality of the product. This must include information on whether the irradiation is for reduction of a bioburden or for sterilisation purposes, and that the irradiation has produced the desired effects. It must be stated whether there are any qualitative or quantitative changes to the product as a result of the irradiation and, if there are, whether these have any significance. Have the changes affected the quality of the product or the potential health and safety of the patient who will use the product? The safety of the irradiated product for the patient is an issue that should be addressed in the quality Expert Report.

Chemistry of active substances (Note for Guidance III/478/87)

The guideline is intended for use by manufacturers who have produced a new active substance that is not the subject of a monograph in a pharmacopoeia (i.e. the PhEur or a pharmacopoeia of one or more of the 25 Member States).

Identity of the material

Full details must be given of the name of the product, plus a description of the material, including its physical form and molecular formula. Its appearance should also be described.

Manufacture

The guideline states that 'a concise but comprehensive account of the manufacture of the active substance should be provided'. This includes the following topics: the manufacturing process; a description of the process; and quality control during synthesis.

Again, the use of flow-charts to illustrate the synthetic process is recommended. All the ingredients used in the synthesis must be described and their quality detailed (e.g. whether they are of pharmacopoeial standard). The controls apply to starting materials and must also indicate the presence of any impurities introduced during the synthetic process. All quality control checks that are carried out at intermediate stages of the process must also be described.

Development chemistry

The structure and chemical and physicochemical properties of the new substance must be described. Considerable importance is attached to being able to fully characterise the chemical structure of the substance, and all the methods used to do so must be fully explained. Again, this information is often required to be supported by the expert in the quality Expert Report. The latest state-of-the-art techniques should be used at all times, ensuring that the data provided are as accurate and clear as possible.

The physicochemical characteristics must be fully described. These include the material's solubility in a variety of solvents, the presence or absence of polymorphism, and its pK_a and pH values.

Regulators are always keen to be made aware of any unusual aspects associated with the compound during analytical development. The precision and accuracy of the tests must be described, and any variation in results produced – which are especially likely in substances of biological origin – must be detailed.

Impurities

The greater the number of ingredients used in the synthetic processes, the greater is the risk of the presence of impurities in the finished product. Impurities can arise from the synthesis itself, from the use of solvents and other materials during purification processes, and from the inevitable presence of degradation products should the active substance be shown to be relatively unstable.

The test procedures used to detect and identify potential impurities must be listed, together with the limits imposed on their presence. A summary of the test results on impurities in batch samples is also required.

Active substance specification

Tests should be carried out to define the specification for the active substance in terms of its physical characteristics, tests for identity, standards for purity and limitation of impurities, and standards and tests for potency. All analytical methods should be described in detail.

Batch analysis

It is vital that the results from routine quality control of the active substance should be presented. Ideally, these results should be from samples which are to be used or are being used in clinical trials and in toxicity tests. The results should include the date of manufacture, the batch size and number, the place of manufacture, the results of analytical tests and the intended use of the batches.

Reference standards

The use of any reference substances for the analytical process should be described.

Radiolabelled product

If the new active substance incorporates a radioactive isotope, all of the above requirements apply.

Requirements in relation to active substances (Note for Guidance III/8315/89)

Classification of active substances

Active substances may be classified as new active substances, existing active substances not included in the PhEur or the pharmacopoeia of a Member State, or an active substance that is included in the PhEur or the pharmacopoeia of a Member State.

New active substances

The requirements for new active substances are defined above in the previous guideline, *Chemistry of active substances*. Information on the new active substance may be supplied by the applicant company or, if it is manufactured by a third party, using the European Drug Master File (DMF) procedure. (For an explanation of the DMF procedure, see below.)

Existing active substances not included in the PhEur or the pharmacopoeia of a Member State

The data requirements are the same as for new active substances, with data supplied either directly by the applicant company or via the DMF procedure.

Pharmacopoeial active substances

These include inorganic substances, vegetable substances and vegetable substance preparations, materials derived from biotechnology processes, organic substances that are extracted from animal or human material, or organic substances that are manufactured or extracted.

Evidence of the suitability of the pharmacopoeial monograph is required in each case. Control of the levels of impurities allowed in the monograph must be justified, and the ways in which the material is prepared must be critically justified by the applicant. The suitability of the monograph must be shown by the applicant to the regulatory authority. A decision tree outlining the selection of the appropriate regulatory procedure for active substances is included in the guideline.

European Drug Master File (DMF) procedure for active substances (Note for Guidance III/5370/93)

This guideline covers both the legal basis for the procedure, and the working of the procedure itself. The DMF procedure can be applied to both human and veterinary medicinal products.

The legal framework

The legal framework for the DMF procedure is based upon the Annex to Directive 75/318/EEC (as amended), and Directive 81/852/EEC (as amended) – Control of starting materials. It applies to active substances not included in the PhEur or the pharmacopoeia of a Member State and to pharmacopoeial active substances. In the latter case, the monograph is deemed inadequate to control the quality of the active substance when it is manufactured by a third party. In this case, a detailed description of the manufacturing method, quality control procedures and process validation must be supplied direct to the regulatory authority by the third-party manufacturer. However, sufficient information about these processes must be given by the third party to the applicant company to allow the applicant company to take full responsibility for the manufactured medicinal product as marketing authorisation holder.

The DMF procedure

The procedure applies to all classes of substances described in the previous guideline. It is the responsibility of the applicant company to ensure that all the information required by the regulatory authority is in fact supplied in the DMF.

Content of the DMF

The content is divided into that supplied by the applicant company, and that supplied by the active substance manufacturer (ASM). However, the ASM must supply the applicant company with sufficient information about the active substance specification for the latter to be able to take responsibility for the material in the approved authorisation.

The ASM provides the applicant's part of a DMF to the applicant directly and it becomes part of the MAA. The ASM Restricted Part is submitted to the regulatory authority alongside the applicant's part.

Information accompanying a DMF

A 'Letter of Access' supplied by the ASM must accompany the DMF to permit the regulatory authority to assess the data in the DMF on behalf of the applicant company. The ASM must also agree to inform the applicant company and the authorities if there are any significant changes to the specification of the active substance which is the subject of the DMF.

Critical appraisal of the DMF documentation

The ASM Restricted Part of the DMF must contain a critical appraisal (validation) of the manufacturing method, batch analysis, and specification and routine tests which have been applied.

Glossary of terms

A brief glossary is included in the guideline.

Use of the DMF procedure

A question and answer guide to the implementation of the DMF procedure is also included in the guideline. This is intended for use by the chemical industry (the primary manufacturer of active substances) and the pharmaceutical industry (the main suppliers of formulations for MAAs).

Impurities in new active substances (Note for Guidance III/5442/95)

The guideline applies only to active substances prepared by chemical synthesis. It does not apply to certain other products, including those generated by biotechnological processes, radiopharmaceuticals, herbal products and products of animal or plant origin.

Classification of impurities

Organic impurities can arise during the manufacturing process and storage of the chemical, and can include materials used or produced at any stage of the manufacturing process (e.g. starting materials, by-products, reagents, ligands and catalysts).

Inorganic impurities also derive from the manufacturing process and can include heavy metals, inorganic salts and filter aids. Residual solvents tend to be well-established materials with known toxicity, and their impurities are usually well characterised.

Rationale for the reporting and control of impurities

This section outlines the information that should be provided by the applicant company about impurities that might arise during synthesis, purification and storage. It should describe those impurities that would be expected from the materials being used, plus the tests that have been carried out to demonstrate their presence/absence, and, if they are present, the limits and quantities applied to those impurities. All impurities present at a level of 0.1% or more must be identified; the same applies to degradation products identified in stability studies at recommended storage conditions.

Pharmacopoeial procedures are often used to detect and quantify inorganic impurities. Limits on the presence of such impurities should similarly be based on pharmacopoeial data. The same criteria apply to the quantification and identification of residual solvents.

Analytical procedures

All analytical procedures for the detection of impurities must be validated and proved suitable for their purpose. Any variation between analytical procedures used during pharmaceutical development and during the commercial manufacture of the product must be explained and justified.

Reporting impurity content of batches

A batch of a medicinal product may be used for (amongst other things) clinical studies, assessment of toxicological data and stability testing. Tabulated data covering impurities in specific batches must be presented. The data should include the batch identity and size, the date and site of manufacture, the manufacturing process used, the individual and total impurity content, the intended use of the batches, and the analytical procedure used to detect the impurities.

Specification limits for impurities

The specification for the new substance should include data on identified and unidentified impurities found during the commercial manufacturing process. Reasons for the inclusion or exclusion of impurities from the specification must be given. This should take into consideration the likely effects – harmful or otherwise – of the impurity.

Qualification of impurities

'Qualification is the process of acquiring and evaluating data which establishes the biological safety of an individual impurity or a given impurity profile at the level(s) specified.' As above, reasons for selecting particular impurities for qualification must be based on safety considerations. When safety and/or clinical studies have been carried out, the level of any impurity is considered 'qualified'. A decision tree is appended to the guideline to determine the action to be taken should the threshold limits for impurities be exceeded. The threshold limits are based upon the maximum daily dose, defined as either less than or equal to, or more than, an intake of 2 g of substance per day.

New impurities

Any change in the manufacturing process may lead to the generation of a completely new, previously absent, impurity. Again, any decision about the identification and detection of the new impurity must be based upon safety considerations.

Glossary

A short glossary explains the terms used in the guideline.

Excipients in the MAA dossier for a medicinal product (Note for Guidance III/3196/91)

Data about the excipients in the formulation must be developed in a similar way to that for the active substance. This guideline refers to specific parts of Volume 2 of *The Rules Governing Medicinal Products in the European Union*,[3] which details data requirements for the active substance. The guideline makes it clear that data in these sections relating to the requirements for active substances must be applied to excipients.

Composition of the medicinal product

Full details of the excipients in the formulation must be given, including their common name, the amount in which they are being used, and the standard of the material being used. Mixtures of excipients must be described qualitatively and quantitatively.

Development pharmaceutics

An explanation of the reasons for the choice of an individual excipient, and the standard of material chosen, must be given.

Excipients

An Annex to the guideline describes examples of different kinds of excipients. The specifications and routine tests applied to an excipient follow the same pattern as for active substances. The specification again depends upon the presence of the material in the PhEur or a pharmacopoeia of an EU Member State, and the scientific data required about the excipient must justify the choice and use of a particular excipient.

If the excipient is well known and has been used in medicinal product formulations for a long time, the properties and characteristics will be clearly defined and the level of scientific data required is correspondingly diminished. However, if the excipient is new, it should in effect be treated in the same way as a new active substance, and the data requirements are the same (i.e. a new MAA is in effect required for the excipient).

The finished product

It is not usually a requirement to carry out identity testing and assays of the excipients in a finished product if all the earlier requirements have been fulfilled.

Plastic primary packaging materials (Note for Guidance III/90/90)

The guideline covers only those plastic packaging materials that come into direct contact with the medicinal product (e.g. a tablet in contact with packaging material in a blister pack). The discussion below refers to the container as the packaging material, although it equally applies to the closure and other parts of the container.

Immediate packaging

A full description must be given of all aspects of the container used as the immediate packaging. Details must include the method of opening; aspects of the design that make the container multidose; and measures taken to ensure that the container is both tamper-resistant and child-resistant.

Development pharmaceutics

The method of administration, the stability of the product, and any method of sterilisation will already have been determined. Reasons for the choice of the container in relation to these issues must be fully given.

Packaging material

A detailed summary is provided in the guideline of the importance of fully characterising the plastic used in the packaging material. It must include details of the technical characteristics of the plastic and any additives in the finished plastic. The manufacturer of the plastic must also be given.

Stability aspects

It is fully recognised by the guideline that plastic materials are inherently unstable and that leaching of ingredients can occur in both directions (both from the finished product into the plastic and from the plastic into the pharmaceutical dosage form). The stability of the finished product in contact with the plastic, in particular if it is not a solid dosage form, must be fully characterised.

Specifications and control tests on the finished product (Note for Guidance III/3324/89)

This document summarises specifications and test procedures, and briefly refers to batch analysis. Appended to the guideline is a glossary of terms used.

Specifications

This guideline is important in that it lists the 'quality' aspects of a medicinal product (see Table 3.4). Other issues addressed include the relationship

Table 3.4 'Quality' characteristics of medicinal products

Note for Guidance III/3324/89 on Specifications and control tests on the finished product

- General characteristics of the pharmaceutical form, particularly pharmaco-technical; that is to say, those characteristics, determined in general by physical tests with limits of acceptance, relating to the product performance or handling (e.g. hardness, friability of a conventional tablet)
- Identification of the active substance(s)
- Assay of active substances (and also for herbal medicines, quantitative determination of the constituents with known therapeutic activity)
- If necessary, identification and assay of the excipients (e.g. identification of colourants used; identification and assay of antimicrobial agents or antioxidant preservatives, with acceptance limits)
- Purity tests (if necessary, the investigation of breakdown products, residual solvents, or other process-related impurities, microbial contamination)
- Pharmaceutical tests (e.g. dissolution)
- Safety tests, including abnormal or specific toxicity tests, where applicable, in particular for biological products

between the specifications referred to in the MAA and those of a pharmacopoeia, and in particular the PhEur; the relationship between the specifications on manufacture (batch release) and at the end of the agreed shelf-life; and the specifications and routine tests used for the batch release of the finished product upon manufacture. Acceptance limits for the specifications are also described.

Test procedures

Reproducibility of data on the medicinal product's specification is very important. Not only should the manufacturer be able to reproduce the data in a reliable way, official laboratories should be able to do so, up to the end of the shelf-life of the product. If applicable, a pharmacopoeial method of analysis can be used. If this does not exist, alternative methods of analysis must be validated against an official pharmacopoeial method.

Batch analysis

This must include the results for all specifications at release, from all sites at which manufacture has taken place.

Impurities in new medicinal products (Note for Guidance CPMP/ICH/282/95)

As previously, this guideline applies to only to chemically synthesised active ingredients. It defines guidance on the content and determination of impurities in a new medicinal product. These are referred to as degradation products. It is in effect an annex to the guideline on Impurities in New Active

Substances (Note for Guidance III/5442/95, see page 42). It applies only to the impurities from the active ingredient(s). It does not apply to excipients, or to impurities which might exist in the product during development.

Analytical procedures

The MAA should include data to demonstrate that the analytical procedures used are suitable for the detection and quantification of degradation products in the finished product. If the analytical procedures used during development are different from those used in commercial manufacture of the medicinal product, the differences should be described and justified.

Rationale for the reporting and control of impurities

Degradation products identified during stability studies conducted under recommended storage conditions should be summarised. If it is not possible to identify a particular degradation product, the data accumulated during the attempt at identification should be included.

Reporting impurity content of batches

The data supplied to show the impurity profile identified in the batch testing of the product are important as an indicator of the quality of the manufacturing process and for determining the expiry date for the product. If impurities are revealed from the testing, their possible origin should be discussed (e.g. by reference to the date and site of manufacture, the batch number and the storage conditions).

Specification limits for impurities

Limits for expected degradation products under predefined storage conditions should be specified. The specification should include the limits for each stated degradation product and the limits for the total degradation products.

'Qualification' of impurities

For a definition of 'Qualification', see page 43. Reference to the decision tree for safety studies (mentioned in the above guideline) should also be made.

New impurities

The degradation profile of a medicinal product may change during pharmaceutical development. If this happens, new degradation products may need to be quantified and identified.

Glossary

Appended to the guideline is a glossary of terms used.

Validation of analytical procedures: methodology (Guideline CPMP/ICH/281/96)

This guideline is a derivative of the *Note for Guidance* on *Validation of analytical procedures: definitions and terminology* (see page 50) and provides guidance and recommendations on how to consider the various characteristics for each analytical procedure. It also indicates the data that should be supplied to support an MAA. The guideline recognises that the analytical procedures used for biological and biotechnological products may be dealt with in ways that differ from those described. The arrangement of the sections in the guideline is itself instructive as to the ways in which the analysis should be carried out.

Specificity

The objective of the analytical procedure will in part determine the way in which specificity is determined during the validation of identification tests, the determination of impurities, and the assay. If it is not possible for an analytical procedure to be specific for a particular chemical, two or more analytical procedures are recommended.

Closely related chemical structures must be identifiable in the analytical validation. It is acceptable for a positive result to be obtained by analysis of a sample containing the analyte compared to analysis of a sample without the analyte.

Assay and impurity tests, usually using chromatographic techniques, must be carried out to determine specificity. If a nonspecific assay is used, additional analysis must be carried out to ensure specificity is demonstrated.

If impurities and/or excipients are present in the material, it must be shown that the analyte and the other components can be separately identified. Reference samples can be 'spiked' with known impurities and/or excipients and the result compared with the actual samples. If impurities are not available, the test results should be compared with another established method (e.g. that cited in a pharmacopoeia). Tests should also be carried out on samples that have been stored or subjected to known stresses (e.g. humidity, light or oxidative conditions).

Linearity

The 'range' of the analytical procedure is given by the limits within which the results from the test can be considered confident (see opposite). There should be a linear relationship across the entire range of the analytical tests. Testing should be carried out on the stock solution of the test substance using a range of concentrations, or on separate weighings of a synthetic mixture of the product ingredients. Statistical analysis of a linear relationship (e.g. calculation of a regression line by the method of least squares) should be carried out. Data from this analysis (e.g. the correlation coefficient, the y-intercept, the slope of the regression line, and the residual sum of squares) and a plot of the analysis should be included in the MAA. A minimum of five concentrations are recommended for determination of linearity.

Range

Closely related to the linearity is the range of results from the analytical procedure. The guideline suggests a number of minimum specified ranges:

- 80–120% of the test concentration for the assay of an active substance or a finished product
- 70–130% of the test concentration for content uniformity for the majority of formulations (exceptions may include metered-dose inhalers)
- for dissolution testing, ±20% over the specified range
- from their reported level to 120% of the specification for impurities (or less if the impurity is especially toxic)
- from their reported level to 120% of the assay specification if a 100% standard is used and the assay and purity test are combined.

Accuracy

The guideline defines the methods of defining accuracy of the assay for active substances and medicinal products and for impurities, and also indicates recommended data for submission.

One method of defining accuracy of the assay of the active substance is by comparing the results with those obtained using a well-established procedure. For a medicinal product, it is possible to determine the accuracy of the assay by applying the same procedure to a predetermined mixture of known concentrations of the ingredients.

The method suggested for determining the accuracy of the assessment of the impurities is to spike samples of the substance or product with known quantities of the impurity. Alternatively, the results can be compared with those obtained from a well-established procedure.

A minimum of nine assays over a minimum of three concentrations that cover the specified range should be used to assess accuracy.

Precision

The precision of the analytical validation is determined by measurement of the repeatability of the tests and their reproducibility. The guideline also specifies the data recommended to be included in the MAA.

Detection limit

The limit of detection can be based upon visual evaluation, upon signal-to-noise (for those analytical procedures that exhibit baseline noise), or upon the standard deviation of the response and the slope. The guideline also states that the method used for determining the detection limit and the actual detection limit itself should be included in the data.

Quantitation limit

Similar approaches to those used for the detection limit should be used for the determination of the quantitation limit.

Robustness

The robustness is a measure of the reliability of the analysis in the event of changes in method parameters. This is expressed as a series of system suitability parameters (e.g. a resolution test) that ensures that the analytical procedure used remains valid throughout any variations. Such variations may include the stability of analytical solutions or extraction time; others may arise in the use of liquid or gas chromatography.

Validation of analytical procedures: definitions and terminology (Guideline CPMP/ICH/381/95)

This guideline provides a collection of terms and their definitions, but states clearly that it is not intended to indicate how analytical validation is to be achieved. It provides a common terminology to replace those previously in use in the three regions involved in the ICH process (the EU, the USA and Japan).

Types of analytical procedures to be validated

The guideline describes the four most commonly used analytical procedures:

- identification tests, used to ensure the identity of an analyte in a sample, commonly using a reference standard against which the sample is analysed
- quantitative and limit tests for the control of impurities
- quantitative tests of the active moiety in samples of substance or formulated product.

As has been described in the previous guideline *Validation of analytical procedures: methodology*, the parameters used in the majority of analytical testing procedures are accuracy, precision, repeatability, intermediate precision, specificity, detection limit, quantitation limit, linearity, range and robustness. Each of these terms is described in the glossary of this guideline. The circumstances when revalidation may be required are also explained (e.g. when there are changes in the synthesis of the active substance, in the medicinal product's formulation, and in the analytical procedure).

Stability testing of new active substances and medicinal products (Guideline CPMP/ICH/380/95)

This document describes the core stability data required to accompany an MAA for *new* active substances and medicinal products. (It does not cover the data that must be submitted in abridged MAAs, clinical trial applications, or variations to approved marketing authorisations; equally, the data required in an MAA for existing active substances and medicinal products are specified in the following guideline.) This guideline states that data generated in one of the three areas that are party to the ICH process (the EU, the USA and Japan) are valid in any of the other two areas.

The primary purposes of the guideline are to explain what data are required to demonstrate that the quality of an active substance or a medicinal product is maintained under a variety of environmental stresses (e.g. temperature, light and humidity), and to determine the recommended storage conditions, re-test periods and shelf-lives.

The data requirements described differ slightly for active substances and for complete medicinal products. A comparison of the two sets of basic requirements stated in the guideline is given in Table 3.5.

General

For an active substance, information on the stability forms a core part of the stability evaluation of the product. The information gained on stability

Table 3.5 Comparison of the primary areas of stability testing required for active substances and medicinal products

	Active substances	Medicinal product
General	✓	✓
Stress testing	✓	✗
Formal studies	✓	✗
Selection of batches	✓	✓
Test procedures and criteria	✓	✓
Specifications	✓	✓
Storage conditions	✓	✓
Testing frequency	✓	✓
Packaging/containers	✓	✓
Evaluation	✓	✓
Statements/labelling	✓	✓

of the active substance is utilised in determining the stability of the formulated final product.

Stress testing

All chemicals are inherently unstable and degrade along predetermined pathways. Stress testing assesses the degree of stability residing in the active ingredient.

Formal studies

The active substance must remain within the predetermined specification limits during its expected shelf-life and the re-test period.

Selection of batches

For active substances, at least three batches must be subjected to accelerated and long-term stability tests of at least 12 months' duration. Equally importantly, the quality of the ingredients used in the manufacture of the active substance must remain the same during initial studies, manufacturing scale-up and the final manufacturing process. This is to permit extrapolation of the stability test results. After the marketing authorisation approval has been granted, the first three production batches of active substance must be placed under long-term stability testing if the results were not available for submission with the MAA.

For the finished medicinal product, the containers and closures to be used in distribution of the product must be the same as those used in the stability tests. The guideline states that 'data on laboratory scale batches is not acceptable as primary stability information'.

Test procedures and criteria

Initial tests on the active substance will have identified the ways in which degradation of the active substance will be most likely (e.g. physical, chemical and/or microbiological). Tests must therefore be selected that most closely monitor those pathways for degradation.

The range of testing on the formulated product is similar, but with particular attention on preservative-efficacy testing and assays on stored samples.

Specification

The active substance used in preclinical and clinical studies will indicate the limits of acceptability of any degradation products. For the finished formulated product, the shelf-life specification must be justified on the basis of changes observed on storage. Upper limits for degradation products must be stated and will be influenced by the changes seen in finished product samples prepared for preclinical and clinical trials.

Storage conditions

For an active substance, confidence is required to ensure that the material remains suitable during storage and subsequent use. Similar storage conditions should be used in storing the active substance and the finished medicinal product. Long-term testing should be carried out at 25°C±2°C and 60%±5% relative humidity (RH) for at least 12 months at the time of submission of the data; accelerated testing should be carried out at 40°C±2°C and 75%±5% RH over at least 6 months. Data from accelerated testing at an intermediate condition may be used to indicate storage stability when the materials are stored outside the label conditions (e.g. on shipment).

Whereas the failure to meet the required specification in accelerated testing is defined as a 'significant change' for the active substance, there are slightly less stringent requirements for the finished medicinal product. A 'significant change' for the finished medicinal product includes: a 5% loss of potency from the initial assay value of a batch; any specified degradation product exceeding its specification limit; the product exceeding its pH limits; or dissolution exceeding the specification limits for 12 tablets or capsules.

Testing frequency

The frequency of testing should be adequate to clearly define the stability characteristics of the active substance or medicinal product. Testing under the defined long-term conditions should take place every 3 months for the first year, every 6 months for the second year, and annually thereafter. For the finished medicinal product, matrixing or bracketing can take place if justified.

Packaging/containers

The actual packaging used in the storage and distribution of the active substance or the finished product should be simulated or be the same as that used in the testing process.

Evaluation

The stability study is intended to ascertain that the active substance and the finished product will remain within defined physical, chemical, microbiological and quality limits when re-tested at predetermined times. One way in which this can be assessed is to 'determine the time at which the one-sided 95% confidence limit for the mean degradation curve intersects the acceptable lower specification limit'. Applying appropriate statistical limits (e.g. p tests) can be beneficial for batches of material where the variability is low.

It may be possible to extrapolate real-time data beyond the observed range in order to define the expiry date at submission of the data, especially if this is supported by the accelerated testing data. However, this must be justified in the submission. Any actions undertaken on the stored finished medicinal product (e.g. reconstitution or dilution) must also be evaluated in the stability testing.

Statements/labelling

It may be possible to state a storage temperature range, which should be based upon the stability evaluation. Specific storage requirements (e.g. 'Do not store at freezing or below') may be applicable. Vague terms (e.g. 'ambient temperature' or 'room temperature') are not to be used.

Stability testing: requirements for new dosage forms (Annex to Guideline CPMP/ICH/380/95)

This *Note for Guidance* is an Annex to the previous guideline, which should be consulted for basic principles. It is very short and merely defines new dosage forms. A new dosage form is defined as a medicinal product that comprises a different pharmaceutical product but contains an active ingredient that is already approved by the regulatory authority. It includes products given by a different route of administration or a new delivery system, or a different dosage form given by the same route of administration. The testing carried out should be based on that used for the parent active substance, although a reduced stability database (e.g. 6 months' accelerated and 6 months' long-term data) may be acceptable when justified.

Photostability testing of new active substances and medicinal products (Guideline CPMP/ICH/279/95)

This *Note for Guidance* is an Annex to the previous guideline, which should be consulted for basic principles. It does not include photostability testing of the product during or after administration.

Light-testing is an integral part of stability testing. All new active substances and new medicinal products should be subjected to light-testing to ensure that unacceptable degradation does not occur. Any changes made to the product require light-testing to be repeated.

Testing should be carried out on the active substance, on the exposed product outside the immediate pack, on the product in the immediate pack and, if necessary, on the product in the marketing pack. The extent of acceptable limits for change of the product is to be defined by the company making the MAA.

The sources of light to be used for testing are recommended in the guideline and include:

- artificial daylight fluorescent lamp
- a metal halide lamp
- a near-ultraviolet fluorescent lamp whose output is between 320 nm and 400 nm.

Samples of the material should be exposed to light that gives not less than 1.2 million lux-hours and an integrated near-UV energy of not less than 200 watts per hour per square metre.

Active substance

There are two elements to the photosensitivity challenge: forced degradation testing and confirmatory testing. For forced degradation studies, simple solutions or suspensions of the active ingredient can be tested in chemically inert and transparent containers. It is possible that the degradation products identified during forced testing would not occur under normal testing conditions. In such instances, if the degradation products are absent from the confirmatory studies, then they do not need to be investigated further. The purpose of confirmatory studies is to ensure that the ideal conditions for handling, packaging and labelling are used.

It is possible to carry out photostability testing of the active substance using only a single batch of the material. If it is clear that the active material is photostable or photolabile, no further tests need be carried out. If the results are equivocal, additional batches should be tested.

Samples are examined at the end of the testing period. Any obvious signs of physical deterioration (e.g. a change in colour, or the development of an opaque solution) should be recorded.

Medicinal product

Tests are carried out in the following order: the fully exposed medicinal product, the product in any intermediate pack, and finally on the packaging to be used for the distribution of the medicinal product. Testing is continued until it is clear that the product is adequately protected from exposure to light. If the immediate pack is clearly impermeable to light (e.g. if it is an aluminium tube), the tests should be carried out only on the directly exposed product.

If a product is to be used in such a way that it will be exposed to light on use (e.g. a skin cream), tests should be carried out to ensure that it is photostable on use. Equally, a product should be tested in such a way that it receives the maximum exposure to the light source (e.g. tablets should be exposed in a single layer).

Samples should be examined to ensure that there have been no gross physical changes. Assay of possible degradation products should also be carried out. For solid oral dosage forms, at least 20 tablets or capsules should be tested. Care must also be taken in sampling from other preparations that may have broken down into nonhomogenous components.

If there have been significant changes in the product, it may be necessary to have special labelling or packaging such that the product remains of an appropriate quality throughout its life.

Quality of prolonged-release oral solid dosage forms (Guideline CPMP/QWP/604/96)

If the therapeutic action is to be prolonged, or attempts are made to reduce possible toxic effects, a formulation may be modified such that the release of active substance is the rate-limiting step in its absorption. Such formulations are described as 'prolonged-release', and the guideline uses this term in preference to the terms 'controlled-release' or 'sustained-release'.

Development pharmaceutics

The reasons for the development of the prolonged-release formulation should be given, along with the pharmacokinetic and physicochemical parameters of the active substance. It should be explained how the prolonged release is to be achieved, whether the formulation is a single disintegrating unit or a multiunit pelletised system, and the release mechanism and kinetics (if known).

In vitro testing using a pharmacopoeial dissolution test should be carried out to determine the release rate of the active substance. Each strength of the prolonged-release product should be tested, and any actions to be undertaken prior to administration by the patient (e.g. if the tablet is to be halved) should also be reflected in the testing procedure. *In vivo* testing will permit determination of the bioavailability of the active ingredient. Correlation of the *in vitro* and *in vivo* testing results should be attempted.

Manufacturing process validation

The details of the manufacturing process should be given that include the critical process parameters. If the validation has been carried out using small-scale batches, the dissolution characteristics of the scaled-up manufacture of the product should be given.

Control tests

A dissolution test is normally included in the finished product specification. This ensures consistent substance release from batch to batch and allows acceptance limits to be set for the dissolution profile during the product's shelf-life. The number of dosage units tested should be stated and at least three points should be determined, including an early one to ensure that all the active ingredient has not been eliminated immediately, and a later point to demonstrate that the majority of the substance has been released. Like all test methods, the dissolution assay should undergo analytical validation, which includes determining the stability of the active substance in solution in the dissolution medium. At least three batches of production scale should be validated, and individual dosage units dissolution test results included.

Stability

The dissolution profile of the active substance must be maintained throughout its proposed shelf-life.

Changes to products

If *in vivo/in vitro* testing correlation has been achieved, minor modifications to the composition of the product or its manufacture may be acceptable without further correlation being obtained. More significant changes usually require the correlation to be reassessed.

References

1. European Commission. *The Rules Governing Medicinal Products in the European Union*, Vol. 3A, *Guidelines: medicinal products for human use: quality and biotechnology*. Luxembourg: European Commission, 1998.
2. European Commission. *The Rules Governing Medicinal Products in the European Union*, Vol. 4, *Good Manufacturing Practices: medicinal products for human and veterinary use*. Luxembourg: European Commission, 1998.
3. European Commission. *The Rules Governing Medicinal Products in the European Union*, Vol. 2, *Notice to Applicants*. Luxembourg: European Commission, 1998.

4

Pharmacotoxicological studies

Safety issues cover all aspects of the preclinical development of a new product. They are covered in Part III of the marketing authorisation application (MAA).[1] In essence, this covers the following:

- toxicity
- reproductive function
- embryo-fetal and perinatal toxicity
- mutagenic potential
- carcinogenic potential
- pharmacodynamics
- pharmacokinetics
- local tolerance
- environment risk assessment.

Mention has already been made in Chapter 1 of the recognition of the importance of trying to limit the use of animals in drug development studies. Nevertheless, studies undertaken on animals are still a requirement of regulatory authorities in assessing the potential beneficial and harmful effects in humans.

To assist applicant companies in the EU to provide the necessary information for each of the above topics, guidelines or *Notes for Guidance* have been produced by the EU Committee for Proprietary Medicinal Products (CPMP) of the European Agency for the Evaluation of Medicinal Products (EMEA). Although the guidelines have no legislative standing, applicants must justify their own processes where they differ from those given in the published guidelines. Adopted and draft EU 'safety' guidelines are listed in Table 4.1. Those that are currently under development within the International Conference on Harmonisation of the Technical Requirements for the Registration of Pharmaceuticals for Human Use (ICH), and which are therefore also to be adopted within the EU, are listed in Table 4.2.

The Safety Working Group has also produced Discussion Papers, Concept Papers and Points to Consider that discuss at greater length than the *Notes for Guidance* particular important issues. Those currently available are listed in Table 4.3.

The guidelines on safety aspects of the MAA are published as a compendium in Volume 3B of *The Rules Governing Medicinal Products in the European Union*.[1] The following summary of safety requirements is based upon the guidelines published in this volume. (The numbering of EU guidelines is convoluted and inconsistent. Later documents, or earlier ones

Table 4.1 Adopted and draft safety guidelines

Guidelines adopted by the Safety Working Party (SWP) of the Committee for Proprietary Medicinal Products (CPMP) of the European Agency for the Evaluation of Medicinal Products (EMEA). Copyright EMEA. Last revised 28 April 2000

Reference number	Title
Adopted guidelines	
CPMP/SWP/2877/00	Note for Guidance on Carcinogenic potential (CPMP adopted July 02)
CPMP/SWP/398/01	Note for Guidance on Photosafety Testing (CPMP adopted June 02)
CPMP/SWP/2145/00	Note for Guidance on Nonclinical local tolerance testing of medicinal products (CPMP adopted Feb. 01)
CPMP/SWP/1042/99	Note for Guidance on Repeated dose toxicity (CPMP adopted July 2000)
CPMP/SWP/997/96	Note for Guidance on Preclinical evaluation of anticancer medicinal products
CPMP/SWP/465/95	Note for Guidance on Preclinical pharmacological and toxicological testing of vaccines (CPMP adopted Dec. 97)
CPMP/SWP/728/95	Replacement of Animal studies by *in vitro* models (CPMP adopted Feb. 97)
Draft guidelines	
CPMP/3097/02	Consultation on Comparability of medicinal products containing biotechnology-derived proteins as drug substance (Released for consultation July 02)
CPMP/SWP/2599/02	Position Paper on the Nonclinical safety studies to support clinical trials, with a single low dose of a compound (Released for consultation June 02)
CPMP/SWP/4446/00	Note for Guidance on Specification limits for residues of metal catalysts (Re-released for consultation June 02)
CPMP/SWP/112/98	Safety Studies for Gene Therapy Products
Concept papers	
CPMP/SWP/160/98	Concept Paper on immunotoxicity revision of the CPMP notes for guidance on repeated-dose toxicity testing and nonclinical local tolerance testing of medicinal products

that have been the subject of revision, are numbered as in Tables 4.1 and 4.2; earlier ones still can only be referenced by their original EU designation. The designation in Volume 3B of the *Rules* is given in the discussion below.)

Single-dose toxicity

This guideline covers the qualitative and quantitative study of toxic phenomena and their occurrence related to time after a single administration of a substance or a combination of substances. The primary use of single-

Table 4.2 ICH adopted and draft safety guidelines

Guidelines which have been developed or which are under development under the auspices of the International Conference on the Harmonisation of the Technical Requirements for the Registration of Pharmaceuticals for Human Use (ICH). Copyright EMEA. Sourced from document CPMP/SWP/2714/99, dated December 1999

Reference number	Title
Adopted guidelines	
CPMP/ICH/539/00 – adopted Nov. 2000	Safety pharmacology studies for human pharmaceuticals
CPMP/ICH/300/95 – adopted Nov. 98	Duration of chronic toxicity testing in animals (rodent and nonrodent toxicity testing)
CPMP/ICH/299/95 – adopted Sept. 97	Carcinogenicity: testing for carcinogenicity of pharmaceuticals
CPMP/ICH/366/96 – adopted Sept. 97	Dose selection for carcinogenicity studies of pharmaceuticals: addition of a limited dose and related notes
CPMP/ICH/174/95 – adopted Sept. 97	Genotoxicity: a standard battery for genotoxicity testing of pharmaceuticals
CPMP/ICH/302/95 – adopted Sept. 97	Preclinical safety evaluation of biotechnology-derived products
CPMP/ICH/141/95 – adopted Sept. 95	Genotoxicity: guidance on specific aspects of regulatory genotoxicity tests for pharmaceuticals
CPMP/ICH/384/95 – adopted Nov. 94	Toxicokinetics: a guidance for assessing systemic exposure in toxicology studies
CPMP/ICH/386/95 – adopted Nov. 94	Reproductive toxicology: detection of toxicity to reproduction for medicinal products (methods: definitions and terminology (CPMP adopted Sept. 93))
CPMP/ICH/385/95 – adopted Nov.94	Pharmacokinetics: guidance for repeated dose tissue distribution studies
CPMP/ICH/136/95 – adopted Dec. 95	Reproductive toxicology: toxicity on male fertility
CPMP/ICH/140/95 – adopted Dec. 95	The need for carcinogenicity studies of pharmaceuticals
Draft guidelines	
CPMP/ICH/423/02 – released for consultation Feb. 02	Safety pharmacology studies for assessing the potential for delayed ventricular repolarization (QT interval prolongation) by human pharmaceuticals

dose toxicity tests in is determining what effects acute overdosage in humans might produce, and by what mechanism(s) death arises. Their use may also assist in designing repeated-dose toxicity studies in animals. The guideline specifically requires that the maximum amount of information be obtained from the minimal number of animals.

Table 4.3 Discussion Papers, Concept Papers and Points to Consider on safety topics

Discussion Papers, Concept Papers and Points to Consider issued by the Safety Working Party (SWP) of the Committee for Proprietary Medicinal Products (CPMP) of the European Agency for the Evaluation of Medicinal Products (EMEA). Copyright EMEA. Situation as at December 2003

Reference number	Title
Discussion papers	
CPMP/SWP/4447/00	Environmental risk assessment of non-genetically modified organisms (non-GMOs) containing medicinal products for human use
Concept papers	
CPMP/SWP/668/02	Development of a CPMP Position Paper on the nonclinical safety studies to support low dose clinical screening studies in humans
CPMP/SWP/3404/01	Development of a CPMP Note for Guidance on the need for preclinical testing of human pharmaceuticals in juvenile animals
CPMP/SWP/373/01	Development of a CPMP Note for Guidance on Risk assessment of medicinal products on human reproductive and development toxicities: from data to labelling
CPMP/SWP/4163/00	Development of a CPMP Points to Consider document on the need for reproductive toxicity studies in the development of human insulin analogues
CPMP/SWP/1053/00	Development of a CPMP Note for Guidance on photosafety testing
CPMP/SWP/781/00	Development of a CPMP Points to Consider document on the nonclinical assessment of the carcinogenic potential of human insulin analogues
Points to consider	
CPMP/SWP/2600/01 Final	Need for assessment of reproductive toxicity of human insulin analogues (CPMP adopted Mar. 02)
CPMP/372/01 Final	Nonclinical assessment of the carcinogenic potential of insulin analogues (CPMP adopted Nov. 01) (Released for consultation Sept. 01)
CPMP/986/96	Assessment of the potential for QT interval prolongation by noncardiovascular medicinal products (of 17 Dec. 97)

Product specification

The finished product and the active substance should ideally have similar impurity profiles. If this is so, the toxicity profiles will also be similar; if it is not, comparative toxicity studies must be undertaken. The physical characteristics of the product's ingredients will be the most likely cause of variations between the finished product and the active substance.

The formulation to be marketed as the finished product should be used in large-animal (e.g. primate) studies. If the pharmaceutical formulation might lead to changes in the bioavailability of the active substance between species, this is particularly important.

As indicated in Chapter 3, when a new excipient is used, toxicity studies must be carried out as if it was a new active substance.

Combinations of substances in finished products (whose use is not normally recommended) require special studies. Each individual substance should be tested, as well as the combination, to exclude any unusual toxic effects.

The active ingredient or finished product might degrade over time. The toxicity of any degradation products must also be determined.

Animals

Equal numbers of both sexes of at least two mammalian species of known strain should be used for single-dose toxicity studies. Qualitative study of toxic signs should be recorded. Qualitative study of toxic signs and quantitative determination of the approximate lethal dose can be done using rodents (e.g. mouse, rat and hamster). To minimise use of animals, failure to find any difference in toxicity between sexes in the first rodent species permits use of only a single sex in the other acute toxicity studies.

Each study should record for each animal used the species, strain, age, sex, weight, origin, whether vaccinated, whether free of specific pathogens and the time spent in the laboratory prior to testing. Details of how the animals are kept, including the amount of water given and the diet, should also be recorded.

Administration

The route and conditions of administration of the substance under test, and the dose given, must be detailed. Two routes of administration are essential, one of which should be the intended use in humans and one to ensure circulatory access. If the intended use in humans is only by intravenous injection, only this route need be tested in animals.

All details of the formulation of administration must be given. If it is not of neutral pH, possible formulation toxic effects must be taken into account.

As wide a dose range as possible should be used to show all toxic effects. The dose–effect range and approximate lethal dose should be determined in rodents.

Observations

Regular observation is essential to track development of any toxicity. The period of observation should usually last 14 days, but may be extended as long as progressive toxic signs are seen.

Autopsy

Some animals will die during the study; others that survive must be killed at the end and their bodies also subjected to autopsy.

Presentation of data

An assessment of morbidity should be given for each species used, at each dose and for each route of administration. Calculations (e.g. of lethal dose) must be fully described.

Repeated-dose toxicity (Note for Guidance CPMP/SWP/1042/99)

For long-term treatment in humans with an active substance, repeated-dose toxicity studies are required. The length of the toxicity study depends upon the anticipated length of treatment in humans (see Table 4.4).

The maximum length of repeated-dose toxicity studies is 6 months. (This has been agreed globally within the ICH process.) This applies even if the treatment is to be continuous, or if the body retains a single dose for a long (unspecified) period. For studies longer than 3 months, 'sub-acute' toxicity studies may be carried out (see below) to determine the dose range for the repeated-dose toxicity studies.

Specifications with regard to the substance and its administration

The finished product and the active substance should ideally have similar impurity profiles. If this is so, the toxicity profiles will also be similar; if it is not, comparative toxicity studies must be undertaken. The physical characteristics of the product's ingredients will be the most likely cause of variations between the finished product and the active substance.

The formulation to be marketed as the finished product should be used in large-animal (e.g. primates) studies. If the pharmaceutical formulation might lead to changes in the bioavailability of the active substance between species, this is particularly important.

When a new excipient is used, toxicity studies must be carried out as if it was a new active substance.

The active substance should be given by the route of administration intended for use in humans. Pharmacokinetic studies should be able to demonstrate how much is absorbed from the site of administration. When it is mixed with food or dissolved in drinking water, demonstration of

Table 4.4 Length of repeated-dose toxicity studies for different lengths of treatment in humans

Proposed length of treatment in humans	Suggested duration of repeated-dose toxicity studies
One or several doses in one day	2 weeks
Repeated doses for up to 7 days	4 weeks
Repeated doses for up to 30 days	3 months
Repeated doses longer than 30 days	6 months

reasonable absorption is necessary. Changes in consumption and growth of the test animal must also be taken into account. If the product is to be given other than orally, any local toxicity at the site of administration must be detected.

The active substance should be given every day unless the rate of elimination is especially slow. If elimination rates are high, dosing more than once a day may be required.

Three ranges of dose should be selected: high, intermediate and low. This will allow demonstration of a range of toxic effects; from organ toxicity at one extreme, to the desired therapeutic effect with minimal toxic effects and blood levels comparable with those expected in humans at the other. Control groups of animals not given the active substance should also be simultaneously tested.

Specifications pertaining to the experimental animal

Pharmacokinetic and metabolic studies in different animal species will indicate which produces a response most similar to that expected in humans. The therapeutic range (the dose range between a therapeutic effect and toxic effects) should be determined.

The choice of species and strain should be justified. Normally, equal numbers of both sexes should be used in the study.

A recurrent problem is choosing the number of animals to be tested. International agreement has dictated that the minimal number of animals to show the required effects should be used. However, there must be sufficient to ensure that all possible toxic effects are seen and that animals can be subject to autopsy during the study without affecting the final statistical analysis. Additionally, there should be sufficient animals that some can be retained after the study to see whether the toxic effects are reversible.

At least two species must be tested, one of which should be a non-rodent. The choice should include a species which produces a response close to that expected in humans.

Animal husbandry

Strict control of the conditions (e.g. the environment and diet) in which the animals are kept is essential. These must be detailed in the study report.

Observations

As mentioned above, all data on test animals must be compared to controls. Accurate baseline data on all physiological, morphological and biochemical values for the control animals are therefore essential. General monitoring on both test and control animals is required throughout the study, including body weight, clinical chemistry, haematology and ophthalmology. Pharmacokinetic parameters and toxic effects will determine the frequency at which monitoring should take place. It is also possible that intake may be affected if the drug is given in the food. There must be compensation for this to ensure that dosing levels are maintained.

Comprehensive autopsy of all animals must take place. The guideline lists those tissues from control animals and those given the high dose that must be histologically examined during the autopsy. Less extensive histopathology is required in rodents: only those tissues that show macroscopic pathological changes need be examined. If only small numbers of other species are used, examinations must be conducted on all tissues from control animals and those given all doses.

Immunointerference

Immunological changes produced by the drug may cause adverse reactions. Even if no immunological are effects expected, those organs most susceptible to such changes (the spleen, thymus and some lymph nodes) must be examined macroscopically and microscopically at the end of the study.

Appendix A to the guideline lists those tissues that must be histologically examined during the autopsy. Appendix B describes the special requirements for drugs that are given by inhalation.

Repeated-dose tissue distribution studies (Note for Guidance CPMP/ICH/385/95)

Pharmacology and toxicology studies can be interpreted more effectively if the absorption, distribution, metabolism and excretion of the active substance are well defined. Usually, single-dose tissue distribution studies are sufficient, but repeated-dose tissue distribution studies may assist in the design of preclinical pharmacology and toxicology studies. However, they are not a general requirement globally, and the guideline therefore explains when they should be considered and how they should be undertaken.

When repeated-dose tissue distribution studies should be used

The following are instances when repeated-dose tissue distribution studies should be considered:

- A single-dose tissue distribution study may indicate that the tissue half-life of the active substance is much longer than that detected in the elimination phase in plasma.
- The plasma steady-state concentration of an active substance or one or more of its metabolites may be much higher than predicted from single-dose kinetic studies.
- If certain tissues show lesions that would not have been expected from short-term toxicity studies.
- When site-specific targeted delivery of the drug is under development.

Design and conduct of repeated-dose tissue distribution studies

All of the previous studies undertaken with the active substance should form the basis for the design and conduct of the repeated-dose tissue distribution studies. When using radiolabelled substances, dose levels, duration of dosage (usually using a minimum of one week), and organs to be examined all need to be considered.

Detection of toxicity to reproduction for medicinal products (Note for Guidance CPMP/ICH/385/95)

All active substances must be tested for potential reproductive toxicity. Tests should be carried out using animals during defined stages of reproduction. For detection of potential long-term reproductive problems, studies over one or two generations of animals may be required. The type of study to be undertaken is determined by: the expected use of the drug product, its formulation and route of administration; the data already collected on toxicity, pharmacodynamics and pharmacokinetics; and the known effects of related compounds.

A range of studies should be undertaken, covering all stages from conception to sexual maturity; observations should also be continued through one complete life-cycle (from conception in one generation to conception in the next generation). The stages in the life-cycle are described in Table 4.5.

Any further studies undertaken to investigate detected effects on reproduction are chosen on a case-by-case basis.

Table 4.5 Stages in the life-cycle for reproductive toxicity testing

Stage	Toxicity effects studied
Premating to conception	Adult male and female reproduction; development and maturation of gametes; mating behaviour; fertilisation
Conception to implantation	Adult male and female reproduction; pre-implantation development; implantation
Implantation to closure of the hard palate	Adult male and female reproduction; embryonic development; major organ formation
Closure of the hard palate to the end of pregnancy	Adult female reproduction; fetal development and growth; organ development and growth
Birth to weaning	Adult female reproduction; neonate adaptation to extrauterine life; pre-weaning development and growth
Weaning to sexual maturity	Post-weaning development and growth; adaptation to independent life; attainment of full sexual function

Animal criteria

The characteristics of animals used in studies must be well defined (e.g. by their health, age, prevalence of any abnormalities and fertility). With the use of young mature adults and virgin females, the animals are likely to be of a similar age and weight.

Mammals should be used, ideally of the same species and strain as used in other toxicological studies. The rodent order of mammals is the most commonly used; in embryotoxicity studies, a second nonrodent mammal (usually the rabbit) is required.

Other test systems are continually being developed (e.g. mammalian and nonmammalian cell systems, both *in vitro* and *in vivo*), but they tend to lack the integrated sophistication of animal studies. They are, however, a useful adjunct and may indirectly reduce the required number of animals.

General recommendation concerning treatment

Dosage selection is critical. The highest dose is selected first based on previous pharmacology, toxicology and pharmacokinetic studies. Lower doses are selected from the higher dose, in intervals based on known toxicity and other factors.

The same route of administration as is to be used in humans should be used. The dose should usually be given once daily but, again, pharmacokinetic data may decrease or increase this frequency.

As with all toxicity studies, control groups employing identical conditions must be used.

Proposed study designs – combination of studies

The most commonly used design is the three-study design to study a combination of effects on:

- fertility and early embryonic development
- pre- and postnatal development, including maternal function
- embryo-fetal development.

Fertility and early embryonic development tests will demonstrate toxicity prior to mating and implantation. In females, this includes effects on the oestrous cycle, tubal transport and implantation; in males, it will show effects on sperm motility and maturation, and on libido). At least one species is used, usually the rat.

Effects on the pregnant and lactating female, and on the development of the fetus and offspring during weaning, will be shown by studies on pre- and postnatal development, including maternal function. In case of delayed toxic effects, observations are continued through to sexual maturity. Adverse effects that might be expected include pre- and postnatal death of offspring, and altered growth and development. At least one species is used, usually the rat.

Studies on embryo-fetal development will demonstrate altered fetal growth and structural changes prior to closure of the hard palate. Two species are normally used: rats and rabbits.

Alternative study designs are accepted in certain cases, which must be individually justified. In a single-study design in rodents, the fertility and early embryonic development stage and pre- and postnatal development stage are combined. A two-study design can be similar, but with mandatory fetal examination. Alternatively, female treatment in the fertility study could be continued until closure of the hard palate (with examination of fetuses), combined with pre- and postnatal development studies. This option uses considerably fewer animals than the above designs.

Statistics

All results must be statistically interpreted, using descriptive statistics (in which the relationship between variables and their distribution is determined) and inferential statistics (establishing the statistical significance of the results).

Data presentation

Individual values for each animal in the study must be clearly tabulated, permitting the history of the animal to be followed from its conception to autopsy. Less frequent positive indications (e.g. of clinical signs and autopsy findings) should be individually grouped in tables.

Testing of medicinal products for their mutagenic potential

The guideline opens with the following definition of mutagenesis:

'Mutagenesis refers to those changes in the genetic material in individuals or cells brought about spontaneously or by chemical or physical means whereby their successors differ in a permanent and heritable way from their predecessors.'

Not only are future generations at risk from genetic changes, the individual taking the chemical is also susceptible to a potential cancer risk.

Objectives of a mutagenicity testing procedure

There are different tests available for mutagenicity detection. The procedure chosen should be of maximum accuracy and of reasonable cost, and be capable of detecting the main types of genetic damage: mutations of genes, chromosomes or genomes. The procedure must also take account of the different organisation of genetic material in prokaryotes and eukaryotes. It should also be recognised that the ability of different organisms and different test systems to metabolise xenobiotic compounds varies greatly. Both *in vitro* and *in vivo* tests must be used in such instances.

Proposed mutagenicity tests for medicinal products

The characteristics of the compound under investigation determine which combination of tests should be used. There are four categories of tests, and one test from each category must usually be used.

The most widely used tests are for gene mutations in bacteria, which are carried out using known and well-characterised bacterial strains. Such tests can detect frameshifts and base-change mutations in DNA.

Tests for chromosomal aberrations in mammalian cells *in vitro* utilise human lymphocytes or mammalian cell lines. Assessment of damage at mitotic metaphase during DNA replication indicates mutagenic potential.

The test for gene mutations in eukaryotic systems can be used both in bacteria and in organisms with complex eukaryotic chromosomal structures. Eukaryotes as complex as fungi and insects may even be used.

Confirmation of the results from the above *in vitro* tests is required by the use of the fourth test, the *in vivo* test for genetic damage. Chromosomal damage is indicated by the bone marrow metaphase and micronucleus tests, and the dominant lethal test. The mouse spot test is widely used.

Interpretation of the results

Extrapolation of the above tests to assessment of potential mutagenic damage in humans is especially difficult. Negative results in all four categories of test may suggest low mutagenic potential. The converse results might indicate a high mutagenic risk. Usually, however, the results produce some positive and some negative results, as a consequence of the different endpoints of the tests. It may therefore be necessary to carry out supplementary tests, whose selection is based upon the intended therapeutic use and the drug's other properties.

Risk/benefit considerations

Consideration of many other factors is necessary in making a risk/benefit assessment of mutagenic potential. These include the pharmacokinetic, metabolic and toxicity profiles; and the intended therapeutic use, the age and reproductive status of the patient, and the intended length of treatment with the medicinal product.

Genotoxicity (Note for Guidance CPMP/ICH/141/95)

This document is an extension of, and in part replaces, some of the above guideline, 'Testing of medicinal products for their mutagenic potential'. In its introduction, explanation is given of the different guidelines currently operational in the EU, in Japan by the Ministry of Health and Welfare, and by the US Food and Drug Administration (which in fact uses for pharmaceuticals the FDA Center for Food Safety and Applied Nutrition guidance). The guideline is highly technical in character, and details:

- specific guidance for *in vitro* tests, covering the base set of strains used in bacterial mutation assays, and the definition of the highest concentration for *in vitro* tests
- specific guidance for *in vivo* tests, detailing acceptable bone marrow tests for the detection of clastogens *in vivo*, and the use of male/female rodents in bone marrow micronucleus tests
- guidance on the evaluation of the *in vitro* and *in vivo* test results.

Explanatory notes, a glossary and (almost unique in such guidelines) a detailed list of references used in the compilation of the text are also included.

Carcinogenic potential (Note for Guidance CPMP/ICH/299/95)

Detection of carcinogenicity is facilitated (but not guaranteed) by almost all known human carcinogens being carcinogenic in experimental animals. However, the converse is not always true, and extrapolating results from animal studies to humans is difficult and sometimes arbitrary. Factors which affect extrapolation include, in humans, the intended use of the compound, the dose, and the route of administration; and in animals, the species tested and the incidence of tumours in specific tissues.

Requirements for carcinogenicity studies

Studies will need to be carried out if the agent is to be administered regularly, either continuously over at least 6 months, or frequently and intermittently such that the amount of drug administered is equivalent to the continuous administration. They are also required when the chemical is related to one of a similar structure of known carcinogenic potential, or where its biological action, long-term toxicity or mutagenic-study results may indicate a potential for carcinogenicity.

Some agents used in the latter stages of terminal disease are themselves carcinogenic in the longer term. However, if the anticipated life expectancy of patients using the medicinal product is shorter than the period in which carcinogenic effects from the drug will develop, carcinogenicity studies are not required. Similarly, insoluble agents which are not systemically absorbed need not be tested in detail for carcinogenicity.

Species and strain selection

Two species should be used in which the metabolism of the compound is known and should preferably be similar to the metabolism expected in humans. Species and strains known to be sensitive to known carcinogens must be used in the studies. Routine use of positive controls is not required. However, the detection of spontaneous tumours in the strains used (but not necessarily in the animals undergoing the testing) should be noted.

Dosage

Anticipated dosage regimens in humans should ideally be used in the studies (with at least daily dosing), and absorption of the substance should be demonstrated. Three dose levels are to be used. The highest dose should generate a minimum toxic effect. This could be target organ toxicity, as shown by organ failure and subsequently identified pathological changes. The lowest dose should be 2–3 times the maximum anticipated human therapeutic dose or pharmacologically effective dose in animal studies. The mean of the high and low doses is chosen as the middle dose.

Practical features

All animals used must be healthy and studies should be started immediately after weaning. They must proceed for 24 months in rats and 18 months in mice or hamsters. A high survival rate may require extension of the study to 30 months in rats and 24 months in mice. Each group must comprise 50 animals, with 50 animals of each sex in the control groups. Provision of a uniform, clearly specified diet throughout the study is essential.

Additional monitoring

Testing must be carried out to ensure maximum determination of carcinogenic data. Any additional data expected to be derived from the studies must not prejudice the primary objective.

Statistical design of the study

All attempts must be made to minimise bias from the study and control groups. This can be as simple as ensuring that one part of the animal house is not environmentally different from another, and can extend to keeping a similar proportion of each group of animals to the main group if the study's start has to be staggered because of the large number of animals undergoing testing.

Terminal investigations

Animals may die during the study or may be killed because they need to be put out of any unnecessary suffering. Similarly, all animals must be sacrificed at the end of the study. Autopsies are essential on all animals, irrespective of the reasons for their decease. Previously discovered toxic effects may suggest particular organs to examine, and determination of the reasons for toxic effects may be assisted by biochemical and haematological studies.

All tissues and organs listed in an Appendix to the guideline must be subject to microscopic examination from all animals given the high dose, and from all control animals. If visible signs of damage are noted, similar examinations are required in the affected tissues. The presence of tumours in any tissues requires the corresponding tissues in the middle- and low-dose animal groups to be similarly examined.

Principles of reporting on carcinogenicity studies

All tumours discovered should be classified according to international definitions (e.g. those produced by the World Health Organization). Raw data presentation should include the number of animals examined and the results of macroscopic and microscopic examination. Results must also include the numbers of animals with tumours, the total number of malignant tumours found in an animal, and the length of survival of each animal.

Analysis of the data

The test results must be assessed as follows:

- total incidence of tumour-bearing animals
- total incidence of tumours
- incidence of tumours involving a specific tissue
- incidence of tumours that are apparently malignant
- latent period to tumour appearance.

Comparison of the results between each of the three dose groups, and between the two control groups, is required. It is also necessary to determine independently any dose-related effects of the substance. The guideline recognises that different studies may need different statistical approaches. Consideration of other factors (e.g. death of study animals from other diseases, and early sacrifice of animals showing clinically detectable tumours) may also require statistical analysis. An increased incidence of tumours in animals receiving the substance compared to control groups is always significant. There may be an increased incidence or reduced latency of malignant tumours, an increased incidence of benign tumours, or local induction of tumours at an injection site.

Use of short-term carcinogenicity studies

The guideline unequivocally states that short-term carcinogenicity studies are no substitute for formal carcinogenicity testing in animals. Positive results from short-term studies always require formal carcinogenicity testing for further development of the substance to a marketable product.

The need for carcinogenicity studies of pharmaceuticals (Note for Guidance EC/ICH/140/95)

The objectives of carcinogenicity studies are to ensure that a chemical does not induce cancer when administered to animals and to extrapolate any such findings to the clinical situation. If any data had been gathered during the early phases of drug development which suggested that cancer could be caused by the new active ingredient, then carcinogenicity studies were required to be carried out. Such studies were especially important for pharmaceuticals expected to be administered regularly for a long period of a patient's lifetime.

Modern techniques have to some extent superseded the carcinogenicity studies in rodents. Currently, genotoxicity studies, toxicokinetics and mechanistic studies are routinely applied in preclinical safety assessment to determine whether 'classical' carcinogenicity studies need to be carried out and the likely relevance of such studies to the use of the chemical in humans.

Historical background

Each of the three regions involved in the International Conference on the Harmonisation of the Technical Requirements for the Registration of Pharmaceuticals for Human Use (the ICH process) had differing stipulations for the carrying out of carcinogenicity studies. If the clinical use was to be continuously for 6 months or more, or there were concerns about the use of a particular agent for less than 6 months, Japan required carcinogenicity studies to be undertaken. In the USA, the requirement for carcinogenicity studies was triggered if use was for 3 months or more. In the EU, administration had to be continuously for at least 6 months, or frequently but discontinuously such that the total exposure was of a similar order.

Objective of the guideline

The guideline lays down conditions for carcinogenicity studies to be carried out with two specific objectives: the avoidance of the unnecessary use of animals in testing; and the consistent application of testing requirements worldwide.

Factors to consider in carcinogenicity testing

The duration of exposure in humans to a clinical agent determines whether carcinogenicity testing should be required (see page 71). Studies are generally needed in certain conditions (e.g. allergic rhinitis, depression, anxiety) for which intermittent but discontinuous treatment is required. Conversely, clinical agents used infrequently or for short periods (e.g. anaesthetics and radiolabelled compounds) do not require carcinogenicity testing unless other studies suggest a cause for concern.

Some chemicals may be a cause for concern about their carcinogenic potential due to their inherent properties:

- they may be in a class of compounds in which other members have shown such potential
- their structure–activity relationship may suggest a risk
- repeated-dose toxicity studies may have generated preneoplastic lesions
- there may be local tissue reactions or other pathophysiological changes caused by long-term retention of the compound or one of its metabolites.

If a compound is known to be genotoxic in one or more other species, it is assumed to be similarly so in humans. If this compound is to be administered over a long period to humans, a chronic toxicity study (of up to 12 months) may need to be carried out to detect any early tumour-producing effects. However, the need for such a study should consider all the available evidence (both *in vitro* and *in vivo*).

It is normal before a marketing authorisation application (MAA) is made for all carcinogenicity studies to have been completed. However, an earlier application, for full-scale clinical trials to be carried out in humans, can be made prior to completion of the rodent carcinogenicity studies if there are no special concerns for the use of the compound in the human population.

If the agent is to be used to treat a serious condition, an MAA can be submitted and approved prior to carcinogenicity study being carried out, especially if there are no suitable alternative therapies available. Where the life-expectancy of the target population is short (e.g. for treatment of advanced systemic cancer patients), long-term carcinogenicity studies may not be required.

The route of administration in the carcinogenicity study in animals should be the same as that intended in clinical use in humans. Even if a different route of administration is used, it should be ensured that all organs likely to be affected by the clinical use in humans are exposed to the agent when given to animals.

Only if there is significant systemic exposure from a topically applied agent (e.g. to the skin or to the eye) may it be necessary for systemic carcinogenicity studies to be carried out. Considerations about the pharmacokinetics, pharmacodynamics and toxicity should be applied to chemically related derivatives of an active agent (e.g. salts, acids or bases of the same active moiety).

Agents that are used as replacement therapy, at physiological levels, and have been produced by either chemical synthesis or recombinant DNA technology do not usually require to undergo carcinogenicity studies. Under other circumstances (e.g. a different patient population, clinical indications or duration of therapy), long-term carcinogenicity studies may be necessary.

Need for additional testing

The occurrence of carcinogenicity in animals cannot always with confidence predict its occurrence in humans. The mode of action of the agent in humans may be different. Mechanistic studies may be beneficial to assess the relevance to human use of findings in animal studies.

Dose selection for carcinogenicity studies of pharmaceuticals (Note for Guidance CPMP/ICH/383/95)

The standard method for the selection of the high dose in carcinogenicity studies has traditionally been the maximally tolerated dose (MTD), which is based upon data from 3 months' toxicity studies. One problem in this technique arises with pharmaceuticals that produce rodent toxicity at low levels: use of the MTD may result in the administration of high multiples of the expected clinical dose. It has been suggested that such high exposures in rodents bear little relationship to the situation that occurs in humans. There may be significant physiological changes in the rodent at such high doses which would not arise in humans at the clinical dose intended. It has traditionally been suggested that the doses selected for rodent bioassays for nongenotoxic pharmaceuticals should permit exposure that:

- allows an adequate safety margin over the human therapeutic exposure
- does not produce major physiological changes or significantly affect animal survival
- is based upon the animal and human dose data already obtained for the agent under test
- makes extrapolation to the clinical situation sensible and possible.

The ICH Expert Working Group on Safety has determined scientifically acceptable criteria for the selection of the high dose in carcinogenicity studies. This has been possible because many of the aspects of the potential use of the pharmaceutical can be predicted: information on the likely patient population is usually known; expected ways in which the pharmaceutical is to be used; and the sort of adverse reactions that will not be tolerated in human use. Any of the following approaches could be used for the endpoints for high dose selection:

- toxicity-based endpoints
- pharmacokinetic endpoints
- saturation of absorption
- pharmacodynamic endpoints
- maximum feasible dose
- additional endpoints.

Determination of the most appropriate endpoint for selecting the high dose for the carcinogenicity study will be based upon all relevant animal data and integration with available human clinical and toxicological data.

It is accepted that the use of rodents to determine possible human carcinogenic potential is not ideal, particularly as the basic mechanisms that lead to cancer are poorly understood. Nevertheless, the following general considerations are important in selection of the high dose for carcinogenicity studies. A limited number of strains of rat and mouse, whose incidence of spontaneous tumours is well controlled, should be used for the studies. Both males and females for all strains and species to be tested in the carcinogenicity bioassay should undergo dose-ranging studies. The anticipated human clinical use of the pharmaceutical should be a determining factor in choosing the carcinogenicity study dose regimen.

Toxicity endpoints in high dose selection

Scientific consensus does not exist for the use of toxicity endpoints other than the MTD. The guideline gives the following definition of the MTD:

'The top dose or maximum tolerated dose is that which is predicted to produce a minimum toxic effect over the course of a carcinogenicity study. Such an effect may be predicted from a 90-day dose range-finding study in which minimal toxicity is observed. Factors to consider are alterations in physiological function which would be predicted to alter the animal's normal life-span or interfere with interpretation of the study. Such factors include: no more than 10% decrease in body weight gain relative to controls; target organ toxicity; significant alterations in clinical pathological parameters.'

Pharmacokinetic endpoints in high dose selection

There is one option for nongenotoxic pharmaceuticals having metabolic profiles that are similar in humans and rodents and low organ toxicity in rodents. An appropriate endpoint for dose selection of carcinogenicity studies may be a systemic exposure that represents a large multiple of the human AUC (area under the curve) at the maximum recommended daily dose.

One problem with this scenario is the likely difference in tissue levels of the pharmaceutical between species despite each having been given the same dose. This may arise through wide variations in metabolism or excretion mechanisms. In such instances, the use of plasma concentrations may be a better guide to dose levels actually achieved. The AUC is thought to be the most accurate pharmacokinetic endpoint as it reflects both the plasma concentration and the length of time it is present in the blood.

Criteria for comparisons of AUC in animals and humans for use in high dose selection

Pharmacokinetic parameters can be used for high dose selection with the following criteria. All aspects of the pharmacokinetic data should be comparable: the strain of rodent used; the route of administration; and the dose range. The changes in pharmacokinetic parameters that occur over time should be reflected by a sufficiently long duration for the pharmacokinetic study. There should be documented evidence of the similarity in the metabolism of the compound in rodents and humans. The relative exposure to the pharmaceutical is estimated following differences in protein binding between species.

Saturation of absorption in high dose selection

Studies to show the maximal absorption of the pharmaceutical by measuring its systemic availability can also be used in selection of the high dose. Similar maximal metabolism and excretion studies can be used to determine the middle and low doses for the carcinogenicity study.

Pharmacodynamic endpoints in high dose selection

The selection of a high dose by use of a pharmacodynamic endpoint can only be done for studies in which a measurable and reproducible response can be observed. The response should also be relevant to the intended use of the pharmaceutical. However, the response should not disturb homeostasis or physiology (e.g. hypotension or inhibition of blood clotting) in a way that might compromise the validity of the study.

Maximum feasible dose

Although, by consensus, the maximum feasible dose is viewed as 5% of the diet, this is currently under review by regulatory authorities. Where a route of administration other than oral is required, issues of practicality and local tolerance will determine the level of the high dose.

Additional endpoints in high dose selection

Alternative endpoints for high dose selection in rodent carcinogenicity studies can be chosen if full scientific justification is given. The middle and low dose selection should be based upon integration of data from human and rodent pharmacokinetic, pharmacodynamic and toxicity studies. Amongst other issues, aspects of human exposure and therapeutic dose, the pharmacodynamic response in rodents, and the unpredictability of the progression of toxicity observed in short-term studies should be considered.

Assessment of systemic exposure in toxicity studies (Note for Guidance CPMP/ICH/384/95)

This *Note for Guidance* explains the basis of the use of toxicokinetics and how to develop testing strategies. It emphasises the need to integrate pharmacokinetic studies into toxicity testing as a mechanism for interpreting toxicology findings and assessing their relevance to clinical safety issues.

Toxicokinetics is an integral part of the nonclinical safety testing programme, allowing attention to be directed towards the kinetics of a new pharmaceutical during the toxicity studies. In doing so, it enhances the value of the toxicology data generated, both in relation to the toxicity tests themselves and in comparing the data with the clinical information generated in human studies. It acts in effect as a bridge between nonclinical and clinical studies. The need for toxicokinetic studies should be based upon a case-by-case assessment of the likely value of such data in preparing an adequate risk and safety profile.

The objectives of toxicokinetics

Toxicokinetics consists of determining the systemic exposure in animals and relating it to the dose level and the time course of the toxicity study. It is also used to relate the levels achieved in the toxicity tests with the observed toxicological findings, and understanding how these might affect the clinical safety of the compound. Furthermore, it will assist in the choice of the species used and the treatment regimen and design of nonclinical toxicity studies.

In toxicokinetics, plasma measurements of the pharmaceutical and/or its metabolites are made over a defined time period. A range of toxicity studies may be supported by toxicokinetics: they include repeated-dose toxicity studies, reproductive studies and carcinogenicity studies. If the route of administration of a pharmaceutical is to be changed, assessment of the implications of the change may be assisted by toxicokinetic studies.

General principles to be considered

It is important that toxicokinetic studies are carefully devised and planned. An assessment of the period of time for which the pharmaceutical has been in the systemic circulation needs to be made. This can be measured using plasma concentrations or by the area under the curve (AUC) of the parent compound or metabolites; less frequently, actual tissue sample concentrations are taken. The selection of relevant dose levels for the animal studies will be based upon the likely exposure and therapeutic dose of the agent in humans. However, it should always be borne in mind that there may be interspecies differences in the pharmacokinetics of the drug.

Dose sampling should be frequent enough to give clear exposure and concentration data, but not so frequent as to distress the test animals. The importance of pre-toxicokinetic studies in assessing the pharmacokinetic profile of the pharmaceutical is clear.

The levels of doses to be given in the study will be based upon the pharmacokinetic and toxicity profiles previously determined. The lowest dose should ideally be one at which no toxic effects are observed. The choice of the high dose level will be determined by the toxicity profile.

It is important that appropriate numbers of animals and dose groups are used for generation of a risk assessment. Toxicokinetic measurements can be made on the entire group of animals undergoing the dosing study or from a selection of the main group under investigation. Ideally, both sexes of animals should be used, unless there is a clear reason for not doing so.

There a number of potential complicating factors in the generation of toxicokinetic data. There may be interspecies differences in protein binding, uptake into tissues and the metabolism of the pharmaceutical. Moreover, metabolites themselves may provoke complicating issues: they may also exert a pharmacological effect and be potentially toxic.

Obviously, toxicokinetic studies should be undertaken using the route of administration that is to be utilised in humans. Planned additions to the routes of administration of a pharmaceutical can affect the safety margin of the product and need to be carefully and fully studied. If there is little difference in the pharmacokinetic profile of the proposed new route of administration compared to previous routes already studied, issues of local toxicity should then be considered and studied.

Detailed statistical evaluation is rarely possible or expected in toxicokinetic studies owing to the relatively small numbers of animals in the studies. There is likely to be a high degree of variation in individual pharmacokinetic results both between study animals and in the same animals in consecutive dosages. Attempts should be made to calculate some mean or median values, although results from individual animals may be just as important in providing a detailed picture of the effects of the pharmaceutical.

Accurate and meaningful toxicokinetic results can only be developed with efficient analytical methodology for the pharmaceutical and its metabolites. Accurate and reproducible measurements of the pharmaceutical and metabolites in whole blood, plasma and serum are essential.

Toxicokinetics in toxicity testing – specific aspects

The following information relates to specific areas of toxicity testing. The frequency of exposure monitoring or profiling may be extended or reduced as required.

Toxicokinetic assessment of single-dose toxicity studies is not usually possible as such studies are often carried out very early in the development process, prior to the development of high-accuracy analytical assay methods in tissues and body fluids. In contrast, toxicokinetic studies should be an integral component of repeated-dose toxicity studies. This is possible once the pharmacokinetic and pharmacodynamic profiles of the pharmaceutical have been determined to a reasonable degree of confidence. Systemic exposure in the species or in the targeted tissue should have been demonstrated in order to generate negative results of *in vivo* genotoxicity studies. For carcinogenicity studies, the treatment schedule should be based upon available pharmacokinetic and toxicokinetic data, usually generated in rat and mouse studies. Toxicokinetic data are especially important when the pharmaceutical is to be administered orally with food.

Toxicokinetic data are not needed for all compounds that are used in reproductive toxicity studies, especially if the relative toxicity in maternal animals is low. However, the data are useful in helping to determine the choice of animal species to be used, the design of the study and the dosing schedule in reproductive toxicity studies. If the pharmacological response to the pharmaceutical is so small as to suggest that systemic levels are not adequate after oral administration, the data from toxicokinetic studies may be helpful in determining the systemic exposure achieved at different stages of the reproductive cycle.

Pharmacokinetic and metabolic studies

It is important to have determined the time course for the absorption, distribution and excretion of a pharmaceutical in relation to its metabolism and its safety. To achieve this, measurements of the compound and its metabolites must be taken in body fluids, tissues and individual organs. It is also important to relate the levels in tissues and other compartments to the level of damage seen in those areas. An assessment must also be made whether the pharmaceutical induces enzyme activity or whether its concentration gradually grows with repeated administration. All such studies should be carried out in animals in which it has been demonstrated that the performance of the drug most closely resembles that in humans.

Substance specification

The physical and chemical properties of the pharmaceutical, including its stability, must be fully characterised. If a radiolabelled substance is to be used in studies, the position of the label is important and must be clearly known, especially in relation to the compound's metabolism.

Methods

Physical, chemical or biological methods can be used to measure body fluid and tissue levels of the drug and its metabolites. Full validation of the specificity, precision, reproducibility and accuracy of all analytical methods must be obtained.

Species

Standard practice dictates that animal species normally used for pharmacological and toxicological studies should also be used for these studies. The reasons for choosing alternative species must be fully explained and justified. Prior pharmacological and toxicological assessment of the pharmaceutical in just a few human subjects may help the choice of animal species for the repeated-dose administration studies.

Drug administration

The route chosen for drug administration should be related wherever possible to that to be used clinically in humans. Extent of absorption should be demonstrated if this is relevant to the likely clinical use.

Presentation of results

Data should be given detailing the absorption and distribution of the pharmaceutical and the time over which this occurs. The blood, plasma or serum half-life should be given, and measurements made of the plasma-protein binding. The major metabolites should be identified and their distribution evaluated. The route(s) of excretion of the pharmaceutical and metabolites must also be determined, including assessment of any enterohepatic recycling that takes place. Overall, quantitative calculation of the fate of the administered dose should be made as thoroughly as is possible.

Nonclinical local tolerance testing (Note for Guidance III/3979/88)

In drug administration, body tissues are placed in contact with what are in effect foreign substances. This *Note for Guidance* is intended to determine whether there are any local adverse effects as a result of administration of the formulated product. Such studies should be carried out prior to dosage in humans.

It may be possible to use *in vitro* tests for local tolerance, so long as the tests have been fully validated as being effective measures of safety of the pharmaceutical.

General considerations for local tolerance testing

The choice of the site of administration is important. A pharmaceutical may come into contact only with tissues at the site, or there may be inevitable or accidental dispersal of the compound to other tissues. The extent of this can largely be predicted: an intravenous route of administration will result in widespread dissemination; topical application will have much more limited distribution, but the possibility of systemic absorption should not be discounted.

If a new pharmaceutical is undergoing testing, it is necessary to determine whether there is any general organ toxicity, for which a route of administration should be chosen that produces some systemic absorption. Only if the pharmaceutical is known to be poorly absorbed, or if it is absorbed but previous studies have demonstrated negligible systemic toxicity, is it deemed unnecessary to carry out further systemic toxicity studies.

Points to consider in the design of local tolerance tests

A number of issues need to be addressed in designing these tests, many of which apply to all toxicity tests. The choice of species is important and will depend upon the particular form of local tolerance being studied.

The proposed clinical use of the pharmaceutical in humans will determine the frequency and duration of administration in animals. It is recommended that the period of administration does not exceed 4 weeks in animals.

If local tolerance is observed (e.g. in the form of lesions), the study should determine whether the lesions are reversible.

The formulation developed for use in clinical studies should be used in the local tolerance tests. This will ensure that the same excipients and vehicles are undergoing testing as in the control groups. Equally, the same dose as that to be used clinically should be selected for the animal studies. Adjustments to the dose may be made by varying the frequency of administration.

As for all studies using animals, it is important that the design of the study ensures maximum results from the use of the smallest possible number of animals. If high levels of adverse and possibly painful effects are seen (e.g. strong irritancy from an application), the test should be terminated at the earliest opportunity.

The route of administration used in animals should reflect that to be used clinically. The route will also determine the dosage levels and the frequency of dosing. It may be possible to use more than one route of administration in a single animal as long as there is no interaction between the different routes, and the degree of systemic toxicity does not preclude this.

Ocular tolerance testing

Testing in eyes is necessary either because the pharmaceutical is to be specifically administered ocularly or because there may be accidental exposure to the eyes (e.g. from shampoos or face lotions). For specific eye preparations single-dose and repeated-dose tolerance testing, usually in rabbits, should be carried out. If the agent may only accidentally come into contact with eyes, single-dose testing is adequate.

In the tolerance test, one eye is studied and the other eye is used as the control. All areas in and around the eye should be examined for at least 72 hours after administration.

Dermal tolerance testing

Such testing is carried out for products intended for administration to the skin, whether they are applied for a local effect or for systemic absorption and effect of the active ingredient. A range of tests is required: a single application; repeated application; determination of sensitising potential; and evaluation of the phototoxic or photosensitisation potential.

The formulation to be used clinically should be used for the local tolerance testing. If the active ingredient is to be absorbed for a systemic effect, variations in the dose may be achieved by changing the amount of product applied or by using a different area of skin.

For a single-dose application, the formulation is applied to shaved or abraded skin (usually in the rabbit). The extent and degree of any adverse reaction (e.g. redness, lesions or scabs) should be monitored for up to 48 hours after application. If these occur, assessment may need to continue for up to 8 days. In repeated-dose studies, the same procedure is followed but with application for a period up to 4 weeks.

The potential of the pharmaceutical to sensitise the skin is usually studied in the guinea pig, following the guidelines for the testing of chemicals.

Parenteral tolerance testing

The route and frequency of administration chosen for the testing will depend upon the intended clinical route and frequency of injection administration (e.g. intravenous, intramuscular or intrathecal).

Observations should be made at the site of injection and in the surrounding tissues for up to 96 hours after injection. Macroscopic and microscopic tissue examination may be necessary.

Rectal and vaginal tolerance testing

Testing on either rats or dogs, a volume of the formulation to be used clinically should be inserted into the rectum or vagina, usually about twice daily for up to 7 days. Gross examination of the local area will reveal any changes in tissue appearance. Faecal examination will indicate loss of blood or mucus; examination of vaginal secretions will permit similar assessment. Full postmortem examination of the local tissue should also take place. Any sensitising potential is usually investigated using guinea pigs.

Preclinical biological safety testing on medicinal products derived from biotechnology

Medicinal products derived from biotechnology are highly complex molecules that need to undergo the same range of preclinical testing as more traditionally chemically synthesised products: pharmacokinetics, pharmacodynamics, acute and chronic toxicity, reproductive toxicity, and carcinogenicity. Such products include hormones, cytokines and other regulatory factors; blood products; monoclonal antibodies; and vaccines. Biochemically, the products can be grouped as:

- polypeptides and proteins shown to be identical to naturally occurring human polypeptides and proteins
- polypeptides and proteins closely related to human polypeptides and proteins but containing known differences in amino acid sequences and/or post-translational modification(s) that may affect biological activity or immunogenicity, or both; this category also includes proteins whose structure may be identical to the natural product but where this cannot yet be verified
- polypeptides and proteins distantly related to or unrelated to human polypeptides and proteins (e.g. murine monoclonal antibodies and viral/bacterial antigens).

A number of issues relating to biological compounds pose particular problems for preclinical testing. Some proteins (e.g. human interferons) are highly specific to humans and are likely to have little pharmacological effect in other species (e.g. rats or dogs). Proteins are composed of amino acid sequences, and the sequence of one protein in humans may be different from that of the corresponding protein in another animal. An adverse immunological response may be precipitated when the compound is given to a dog that would not arise in humans.

This *Note for Guidance* gives general advice on the safety tests and their use for all biotechnology-derived products and then goes on to discuss specific guidance for each of the product groups described above.

Safety tests for biotechnology-derived products

The need for flexibility and the use of a wide range of investigations in preclinical testing is stressed in this *Note for Guidance*. Because of the biological nature of the material and the nature of biological production, there are also problems in the reproducibility of batch manufacture and the determination of the purity of batch production. There must be extremely high levels of quality assurance and Good Manufacturing Practice procedures for such naturally occurring pharmaceutical products.

As described above, the selection of a species for preclinical testing can pose problems. Immunoreactivity studies need to have been carried out and species-specific pharmacological effects identified prior to starting preclinical testing. Where a particular species has proved acceptable to use with one group of biotechnology-derived products, it is likely that a new member of that group can also be appropriately used in the same species.

The planned clinical use of the pharmaceutical will be a guide to the selection of doses for preclinical studies. Dose–target organ toxicity should be studied using a range of increasing doses. Where there are differences in the pharmacological response between humans and the test species, this should be reflected in the range of doses selected.

Some biological products administered have only a very short half-life and/or are given in only very small quantities (e.g. vaccines). Classical pharmacokinetic studies of absorption, distribution, metabolism and excretion may therefore not be feasible. Instead, an assessment of the pharmacokinetic profile, including measurement of the active entity over time and the time over which the pharmacological effect is seen, should be performed very early in the development phase.

Pharmacodynamic testing includes the assessment of likely indications for the product and potential drug interactions. Such testing is carried out with biotechnology-derived products in a similar way to that used for chemically synthesised compounds. Dose–response relationships need to be determined using likely therapeutic doses. Assessment is also carried out at higher dose levels to see whether any adverse effects are seen on body tissues at these levels.

Toxicological studies must take into account the potential differences between the response in humans and that in animals. As such, the range of tests used is identical to that used for chemical compounds: single-dose toxicity, repeated-dose toxicity, local tolerance, reproductive toxicity and assessment of a potential mutagenic and/or carcinogenic effect. It is likely to be in the latter tests for mutagenicity and carcinogenicity that most difficulties will arise for products derived from biotechnology.

Short-term tests for measuring any potential mutagenic and carcinogenic effects are dependent upon the availability of sufficiently sensitive analytical methods to measure the identity, quality and purity of the product. Long-term tests are only valid if a potential for carcinogenic effects might be predicted from the biological action of the product or if the product has demonstrated significant levels of accumulation (through a lack of metabolism or excretion) in previous studies.

It is almost inevitable that a biological compound will generate effects on the immune system – indeed, that is the way in which some exert their pharmacological effects (e.g. cytokines). What is more difficult to assess is the importance of such effects for the potential toxicity of the product, especially if it induces the formation of antibodies and immune-complexes. An investigation of the timescale for the formation of antibodies and immune-complexes should be undertaken, if feasible, and of whether the product interacts with the immune system cells, causing their dysfunction.

Safety testing – hormones, cytokines and other regulatory factors

These agents are defined as 'secreted, nonantibody, soluble mediators of cellular function or behaviour'. They include:

- endocrine products (e.g. insulin, growth hormone)
- growth factors (e.g. erythropoietin and epidermal growth factor)
- antiviral cytokines
- lymphokines and monokines
- cytotoxins
- other regulatory factors.

For blood products (e.g. albumins, complement components and blood-clotting enzymes), comparison of the rDNA-derived blood products with naturally occurring examples is recommended. Extensive safety testing, beyond pharmacokinetic studies and toxicological measurements, is not usually required.

The testing of monoclonal antibodies includes pharmacodynamic measurements that demonstrate pharmacological activity in a range of body systems. Studies should ensure that there is no unwanted binding of the monoclonal antibodies to various human tissues. More extensive studies (e.g. reproductive toxicity and local effects) should be carried out only if they relate to the intended clinical use, and are determined on a case-by-case basis.

References

1. European Commission. *The Rules Governing Medicinal Products in the European Union*, Vol. 3B, *Guidelines: medicinal products for human use: safety, environment and information*. Luxembourg: European Commission, 1998.

5

Clinical studies

Efficacy issues deal with all aspects of the clinical development of a new product. They are covered in Part IV of the marketing authorisation application (MAA). In essence, this covers the following:

- pharmacodynamics
- pharmacokinetics
- clinical trials
- post-marketing experience (if available)
- published and unpublished experience.

To assist applicant companies in the EU provide the necessary information for each of the above topics, guidelines or *Notes for Guidance* have been produced by the EU Committee for Proprietary Medicinal Products (CPMP) of the European Agency for the Evaluation of Medicinal Products (EMEA). Although the guidelines have no legislative standing, applicants must justify their own processes where they differ from those given in the published guidelines. Adopted and draft EU 'efficacy' guidelines are listed in Table 5.1. Those that are currently under development within the International Conference on Harmonisation of the Technical Requirements for the Registration of Pharmaceuticals for Human Use (ICH) and which are therefore also to be adopted within the EU, are listed in Table 5.2.

The Efficacy Working Group of the CPMP has also produced Concept Papers and Points to Consider documents that discuss particular important issues at greater length than the *Notes for Guidance*. Those currently available are listed in Tables 5.3 and 5.4.

The guidelines on efficacy aspects of the MAA are published as a compendium in Volume 3C of *The Rules Governing Medicinal Products in the European Union*[1].

Good Clinical Practice (GCP) (Guideline CPMP/ICH/135/95)

A minimum standard has been set for the performance of clinical trials that involve human subjects. Good Clinical Practice (GCP) ensures the validity of clinical trial data and covers the design, conduct, recording and reporting of clinical trials. It also ensures that the rights, welfare and safety of subjects involved in trials are maintained and are consistent with the principles stated in the World Medical Association Declaration of Helsinki,

Table 5.1 Adopted and draft efficacy guidelines

Guidelines proposed and adopted by the Efficacy Working Party (EWP) of the Committee for Proprietary Medicinal Products (CPMP) of the European Agency for the Evaluation of Medicinal Products (EMEA). Copyright EMEA. Situation as at December 2003

Reference number	Title
Adopted guidelines	
CPMP/EWP/205/95 Revision 2	Note for Guidance on Evaluation of anticancer medicinal products in man (CPMP adopted Sept. 02)
CPMP/EWP/282/02	Position paper on the Regulatory requirements for the authorisation of low-dose modified release formulations in the secondary prevention of cardiovascular events (final)
CPMP/EWP/1080/00	Note for Guidance on Clinical investigation of medicinal products in the treatment of diabetes mellitus (CPMP adopted May 02)
CPMP/EWP/518/97 Revision 1	Note for Guidance on Clinical investigation of medicinal products in the treatment of depression (CPMP adopted Apr. 02)
CPMP/EWP/714/98 Revision 1	Note for Guidance on the Clinical investigation of medicinal products in the treatment of peripheral arterial occlusive disease (CPMP adopted Apr. 02)
CPMP/180/95	Guideline for PMS studies for metered dose inhalers with new propellants
CPMP/EWP/2747/00	Note for Guidance on Coordinating investigator signature of clinical study reports (Adopted Oct. 01)
CPMP/EWP/561/98	Note for Guidance on Clinical investigation of medicinal products for the treatment of multiple sclerosis (Adopted July 01)
CPMP/EWP/QWP/1401/98	Note for Guidance on the Investigation of bioavailability and bioequivalence (Adopted July 01)
CPMP/EWP/567/98	Note for Guidance on Clinical investigation of medicinal products for bipolar disorder (CPMP adopted Apr. 01)
CPMP/EWP/552/95 Revision 1	Note for Guidance on Post-menopausal osteoporosis in women (CPMP adopted Jan. 01)
CPMP/EWP/566/98 Revision 1	Note for Guidance on Clinical investigation of medicinal products in the treatment of epileptic disorders (CPMP adopted Nov. 2000)
CPMP/EWP/519/98	Note for Guidance on Clinical investigation of steroid contraceptives in women
CPMP/EWP/235/95 Revision 1	Revision 1 Note for Guidance on the clinical investigation of medicinal products in the treatment of cardiac failure (CPMP adopted Dec. 99)
CPMP/EWP/563/98	Note for Guidance on Clinical Investigation of medicinal products for the treatment of venous thromboembolic disease (CPMP adopted Dec. 99)
CPMP/EWP/280/96	Note for Guidance on Modified release oral and transdermal dosage forms: Section II (pharmacokinetic and clinical evaluation)
CPMP/EWP/463/97	Note for guidance on Clinical evaluation of new vaccines
CPMP/EWP/563/95	Note for guidance on Clinical investigation of medicinal products in the treatment of Parkinson's disease
CPMP/EWP/238/95 Revision 1	Note for Guidance on Clinical investigation on medicinal products in the treatment of hypertension (CPMP adopted May 97, revised Nov. 98)

continued

Table 5.1 Adopted and draft efficacy guidelines (*cont.*)

Reference number	Title
CPMP/EWP/559/95	Note for guidance on the Clinical investigation of medicinal products in the treatment of schizophrenia (CPMP adopted Feb. 98)
CPMP/EWP/281/96	Note for Guidance on the Clinical investigation of drugs used for weight control (CPMP adopted Dec. 97)
CPMP/EWP/560/95	Note for Guidance on the Investigation of drug interactions (CPMP adopted Dec. 97)
CPMP/EWP/553/95	Note for Guidance on Medicinal products in the treatment of Alzheimer's disease (CPMP adopted July 97)
CPMP/EWP/520/96	Note for Guidance on the Pharmacodynamic section of the SPC for antibacterial medicinal products (CPMP adopted June 97)
CPMP/EWP/234/95	Note for guidance on the Clinical investigation of anti-anginal medicinal products in stable angina pectoris
CPMP/EWP/558/95	Note for Guidance on Evaluation of new antibacterial medicinal products (CPMP adopted Apr. 97)
CPMP/EWP/462/95	Note for Guidance on Clinical investigation of medicinal products in children (CPMP adopted Mar. 97)
CPMP/EWP/240/95	Note for Guidance on Fixed combination medicinal products (CPMP adopted Apr. 96)
CPMP/EWP/555/95	Note for Guidance on Clinical trials with haematopoietic growth factors for the prophylaxis of infection following myelosuppressive or myeloablative therapy (CPMP adopted Mar. 96)
CPMP/EWP/237/95	Note for Guidance on Antiarrhythmics (CPMP adopted Nov. 95)
CPMP/EWP/239/95	Note for Guidance on the Clinical requirements for locally applied, locally acting products containing known constituents (CPMP adopted Nov. 95)
Draft guidelines	
CPMP/EWP/788/01	Note for Guidance on the Clinical investigation of medicinal products for treatment of migraine (Released for consultation Sept. 02)
CPMP/3097/02	Consultation Note for Guidance on Comparability of medicinal products containing biotechnology-derived proteins as drug substance (Released for consultation July 02)
CPMP/EWP/633/02	Clinical development of medicinal products for the treatment of HIV infection (Released for consultation July 02)
CPMP/EWP/49/01	Appendix to the CPMP Note for Guidance on the Clinical investigation of medicinal products in the treatment of schizophrenia, on the methodology of clinical trials concerning the development of depot preparations of approved medicinal products in schizophrenia (Released for consultation Feb. 02)
CPMP/EWP/18/01	Note for Guidance on the Clinical investigation of medicinal products in the treatment of urinary incontinence in women (Released for consultation Nov. 01)
CPMP/EWP/2922/00	Note for Guidance on the Clinical investigation of medicinal products in the treatment of asthma (Released for consultation Nov. 01)
CPMP/EWP/612/00	Note for Guidance on the Clinical investigation of medicinal products for treatment of pain (Released for consultation Nov. 01)

Table 5.2 ICH adopted and draft efficacy guidelines

Guidelines which have been developed or which are under development under the auspices of the International Conference on the Harmonisation of the Technical Requirements for the Registration of Pharmaceuticals for Human Use (ICH). Situation as at December 2003

Reference number	Title
Adopted guidelines	
CPMP/ICH/287/95 – modification released for information Nov. 2000	Clinical safety data management: data elements for transmission of individual case safety reports (ICH ICSR DTD Version 2.3)
CPMP/ICH/2711/99 – adopted July 2000	Clinical investigation of medicinal products in the paediatric population
CPMP/ICH/364/96 – adopted July 2000	Choice of control group for clinical trials
CPMP/ICH/363/96 – adopted Mar. 98	Statistical principles for clinical trials
CPMP/ICH/289/95 – adopted Mar. 98	Ethnic factors in the acceptability of foreign clinical data
CPMP/ICH/291/95 – adopted Sept. 97	General considerations for clinical trials
CPMP/ICH/135/95 – adopted July 96	Good Clinical Practice
CPMP/ICH/288/95 – adopted Dec. 96	Clinical safety data management: periodic safety update reports for marketed drugs
CPMP/ICH/377/95 – adopted Nov. 94	Good clinical safety data management: definitions and standards for expedited reporting
CPMP/ICH/375/95 – adopted Nov. 94	Population exposure: the extent of population exposure to assess clinical safety
CPMP/ICH/378/95 – adopted May 94	Dose response information to support drug registration
CPMP/ICH/379/95 – adopted Sept. 93	Studies in support of special populations: geriatrics
CPMP/ICH/137/95 – adopted Dec. 95	Structure and content of clinical study reports (Annexes I, II, III, IVa, IVb, V, VI, VII and VIII)
Draft guidelines	
CPMP/ICH/4679/02 – released for consultation Sept. 02	Clinical safety data management periodic safety update reports for marketed drugs
CPMP/ICH/541/00 – released for consultation June 2000	Principles for clinical evaluation of new antihypertensive drugs

entitled 'Ethical Principles for Medical Research Involving Human Subjects' (for the complete text of the Declaration, see Appendix 2).

This guideline was developed under the auspices of the International Conference on the Harmonisation of the Technical Requirements for the Registration of Pharmaceuticals for Human Use (ICH process), and is applicable in the EU, the USA and Japan. Clinical trial data that have been developed according to this guideline should therefore be acceptable by regulatory authorities in each of the three regions, together with Australia, Canada, Nordic countries and the World Health Organization (WHO), who were also involved in its development.

Table 5.3 Efficacy Concept Papers

Concept Papers adopted by the Efficacy Working Party (EWP) of the Committee for Proprietary Medicinal Products (CPMP) of the European Agency for the Evaluation of Medicinal Products (EMEA). Copyright EMEA. Situation as at December 2003

Reference number	Title
CPMP/EWP/2459/02	CPMP Points to Consider on Methodological issues in confirmatory clinical trials with flexible design and analysis plan
CPMP/EWP/2339/02	CPMP Note for Guidance on Evaluation of the pharmacokinetics of medicinal products in patients with hepatic impairment
CPMP/EWP/2454/02	CPMP Note for Guidance on Clinical investigation of medicinal products ot the treatment of psoriasis
CPMP/EWP/2455/02	CPMP Points to Consider on Allergic rhinoconjunctivitis
CPMP/EWP/968/02	CPMP Points to Consider on the Evaluation of the pharmacokinetics of medicinal products in the paediatric population
CPMP/EWP/226/02	CPMP Note for Guidance on the Clinical pharmacokinetic investigation of the pharmacokinetics of peptides and proteins
CPMP/EWP/225/02	CPMP Note for Guidance on the Evaluation of the pharmacokinetics of medicinal products in patients with impaired renal function
CPMP/EWP/1412/01	Revision of the CPMP Note for Guidance on Evaluation of new antibacterial medicinal products (CPMP/EWP/558/95) and the CPMP Note for Guidance on the pharmacodynamic section of the SPC for antibacterial medicinal products (CPMP/EWP/520/96)
CPMP/EWP/2991/01	Addendum on the Clinical requirements of modified release medicinal products submitted as a line extension of an existing marketing authorisation to the CPMP Note for Guidance on modified release oral and transdermal dosage forms: Section II (pharmacokinetic and clinical evaluation) (CPMP/EWP/280/96)
CPMP/EWP/1533/01	Addendum on Acute cardiac failure to the CPMP Note for Guidance on clinical investigation of medicinal products in the treatment of acute cardiac failure
CPMP/EWP/PHVWP/1417/01	CPMP Note for Guidance on the Use of medicinal products during pregnancy: need for post-marketing data
CPMP/EWP/512/01	CPMP Note for Guidance on the Evaluation of medicinal products for the treatment of dyslipoproteinaemia
CPMP/EWP/967/01	CPMP Note for Guidance on the Evaluation of medicinal products indicated for thrombolysis in acute myocardial infarction (AMI)
CPMP/EWP/2158/99	CPMP Points to Consider on Biostatistical/methodological issues arising from recent. CPMP discussions on licensing applications: choice of delta

Table 5.4 Efficacy Points to Consider

Points to Consider adopted by the Efficacy Working Party (EWP) of the Committee for Proprietary Medicinal Products (CPMP) of the European Agency for the Evaluation of Medicinal Products (EMEA). Copyright EMEA. Situation as at December 2003

Reference number	Title
CPMP/EWP/908/99	Multiplicity issues in clinical trials (CPMP adopted Sept. 02)
CPMP/EWP/1343/01	New antifungal agents for invasive fungal infections (Released for consultation July 02)
CPMP/EWP/785/97	Evaluation of medicinal products for the treatment of irritable bowel syndrome (Released for consultation Apr. 02)
CPMP/602/95 Rev. 3	Assessment of anti-HIV medicinal products (Adopted by CPMP Dec. 01)
CPMP/EWP/4151/00	Requirements for clinical documentation for metered dose inhalers (MDI) (Released for consultation Jan. 02)
CPMP/EWP/2863/99	Adjustment for baseline covariates (Released for consultation Dec. 01)
CPMP/EWP/1776/99	Missing data (Adopted Nov. 01)
CPMP/EWP/1119/98	Evaluation of diagnostic agents (Adopted Nov. 01)
CPMP/EWP/560/98	Clinical investigation of medicinal products for the treatment of acute stroke (Adopted Sept. 01)
CPMP/EWP/908/99	Biostatistical/methodological issues arising from recent CPMP discussions on licensing applications: adjustment for multiplicity and related topics (Released for consultation July 01)
CPMP/EWP/2284/99	Clinical investigation of medicinal products for the management of Crohn's disease (Adopted by CPMP June 01)
CPMP/2330/99	Application with (1) Meta-analyses and (2) One pivotal study (Adopted by CPMP May 01)
CPMP/EWP/565/98	Clinical investigation of medicinal products for the treatment of amyotrophic lateral sclerosis (Adopted Oct. 2000)
CPMP/EWP/482/99	Switching between superiority and noninferiority (Adopted July 2000)
CPMP/EWP/2655/99	Pharmacokinetics and pharmacodynamics in the development of antibacterial medicinal products (Adopted July 2000)
CPMP/EWP/707/98	Clinical investigation of medicinal products for the prophylaxis of intra- and postoperative venous thromboembolic risk (CPMP approved June 2000)
CPMP/EWP/570/98	Clinical investigation of new medicinal products for the treatment of acute coronary syndrome (ACS) without persistent ST-segment elevation
CPMP/EWP/197/99	Endpoints in clinical studies with haematopoietic growth factors for mobilisation of autologous stem cells
CPMP/EWP/863/98	Wording of *Helicobacter pylori* eradication therapy in selected SPC sections
CPMP/EWP/562/98	Clinical investigation of medicinal products in the treatment of patients with chronic obstructive pulmonary disease (COPD)
CPMP/EWP/556/95	Clinical investigation of slow-acting antirheumatic medicinal products in rheumatoid arthritis
CPMP/EWP/784/97	Clinical investigation of medicinal products used in the treatment of osteoarthritis
CPMP/EWP/021/97	Hormone replacement therapy (Nov. 97)
CPMP/EWP/504/97	Clinical investigation of medicinal products in the treatment of patients with acute respiratory distress syndrome (Oct. 97)

continued

Table 5.4 Efficacy Points to Consider (*cont.*)

Reference number	Title
CPMP/EWP/556/95	Clinical investigation of slow-acting antirheumatic medicinal products in rheumatoid arthritis
CPMP/EWP/784/97	Clinical investigation of medicinal products used in the treatment of osteoarthritis
CPMP/EWP/021/97	Hormone replacement therapy (Nov. 97)
CPMP/EWP/504/97	Clinical investigation of medicinal products in the treatment of patients with acute respiratory distress syndrome (Oct. 97)

A comprehensive glossary of terms used in the conduct of clinical trials is given in the guideline (see Table 5.5).

The principles of ICH Good Clinical Practice

The basis for conducting a clinical trial is that there must be some likely benefit from doing so and that any potential risks associated with the trial are outweighed by the potential benefits. A trial should not be conducted with the advancement of science as the sole objective; the rights, well-being and safety of trial subjects are the paramount considerations.

Preclinical studies

Sufficient preclinical studies should have been carried out, covering both clinical and nonclinical aspects of the medicinal product under investigation, to understand what the expected effects of the product will be. The most important document for a clinical trial is the protocol: this must have been approved by the institutional review board (IRB)/independent ethics committee (IEC). (For convenience, the term IEC will be used in the discussion below.)

Medical care

Participants in the trial must be under the medical care of a qualified physician (or where appropriate a qualified dentist) whose training, education and experience must be adequate for the task assigned. Each subject must have indicated that they have freely given informed consent to participate in the trial.

Records

Accurate recording, analysis and auditing of all clinical trial information is vital. Records that might identify subjects must be handled to maintain full confidentiality, and in accordance with all current regulatory requirements.

Table 5.5 Glossary of terms used in the conduct of clinical trials

Term	Definition
Adverse drug reaction (ADR)	In the preapproval clinical experience with a new medicinal product or its new usages, particularly as the therapeutic dose(s) may not be established: all noxious and unintended responses to a medicinal product related to any dose should be considered adverse drug reactions. The phrase 'responses to a medicinal product' means that a causal relationship between a medicinal product and an adverse event is at least a reasonable possibility (i.e. the relationship cannot be ruled out).
	Regarding marketed medicinal products: a response to a drug which is noxious and unintended and which occurs at doses normally used in man for prophylaxis, diagnosis or therapy of diseases or for modification of physiological function (see Note for Guidance on Clinical safety data management: definitions and standards for expedited reporting).
Adverse event (AE)	Any untoward medical occurrence in a patient or clinical investigation subject administered a pharmaceutical product and which does not necessarily have a causal relationship with this treatment. An adverse event (AE) can therefore be any unfavourable and unintended sign (including an abnormal laboratory finding), symptom or disease temporally associated with the use of a medicinal (investigational) product, whether or not related to the medicinal (investigational) product (see Note for Guidance on Clinical safety data management: definitions and standards for expedited reporting).
Applicable regulatory requirements	Any law(s) and regulation(s) addressing the conduct of clinical trials of investigational products.
Approval (in relation to Institutional Review Boards)	The affirmative decision of the Institutional Review Board (IRB) that the clinical trial has been reviewed and may be conducted at the institution site within the constraints set forth by the IRB, the institution, Good Clinical Practice (GCP), and the applicable regulatory requirement(s).
Audit	A systematic and independent examination of trial-related activities and documents to determine whether the evaluated trial-related activities were conducted, and the data were recorded, analysed and accurately reported according to the protocol, sponsor's standard operating procedures (SOPs), Good Clinical Practice (GCP) and the applicable regulatory requirement(s).
Audit certificate	A declaration of confirmation by the auditor that an audit has taken place.
Audit report	A written evaluation by the sponsor's auditor of the results of the audit.
Audit trail	Documentation that allows reconstruction of the course of events.

continued

Table 5.5 Glossary of terms used in the conduct of clinical trials (*cont.*)

Term	Definition
Blinding/masking	A procedure in which one or more of the parties to the trial are kept unaware of the treatment assignments(s). Single-blinding usually refers to the subject(s) being unaware; double-blinding usually refers to the subject(s), investigator(s), monitor and, in some cases, data analyst(s) being unaware of the treatment assignment(s).
Case Report Form (CRF)	A printed, optical or electronic document designed to record all of the protocol required information to be reported to the sponsor on each trial subject.
Clinical trial/study	Any investigation in human subjects intended to discover or verify the clinical, pharmacological, and/or other pharmacodynamic effects of an investigational products(s), and/or to identify any adverse reactions to an investigational product(s), and/or to study absorption, distribution, metabolism and excretion of an investigational product(s) with the object of ascertaining its safety and/or efficacy. The terms 'clinical trial' and 'clinical study' are synonymous.
Clinical trial/study report	A written description of a trial/study of any therapeutic, prophylactic or diagnostic agent conducted in human subjects, in which the clinical and statistical description, presentations and analyses are fully integrated into a single report (see Note for Guidance on Structure and content of clinical study reports).
Comparator (product)	An investigational or marketed product (i.e. active control), or placebo, used as a reference in a clinical trial.
Compliance (in relation to trials)	Adherence to all the trial-related requirements, Good Clinical Practice (GCP) and the applicable regulatory requirement(s).
Confidentiality	Prevention of disclosure, to other than authorised individuals, or a sponsor's proprietary information or a subject's identity.
Contract	A written, dated and signed agreement between two or more involved parties that sets out any arrangements on delegation and distribution of tasks and obligations and, if appropriate, on financial matters. The protocol may serve as a basis of a contract.
Coordinating Committee	A committee that a sponsor may organise to coordinate the conduct of a multicentre trial.
Coordinating investigator	An investigator assigned the responsibility for the coordination of investigators at different centres participating in a multicentre trial.
Contract Research Organisation (CRO)	A person or organisation (commercial, academic or other) contracted by the sponsor to perform one or more of a sponsor's trial-related duties and functions.

continued

Table 5.5 Glossary of terms used in the conduct of clinical trials (*cont.*)

Term	Definition
Direct access	Permission to examine, analyse, verify and reproduce any records and reports that are important to evaluation of a clinical trial. Any party (e.g. domestic and foreign regulatory authorities, sponsor's monitors and auditors) with direct access should take all reasonable precautions within the constraints of the applicable regulatory requirement(s) to maintain the confidentiality of subjects' identities and sponsor's proprietary information.
Documentation	All records, in any form (including but not limited to written, electronic, magnetic and optical records, and scans, radiographs and electrocardiograms) that describe or record the methods, conduct, and/or results of a trial, the factors affecting a trial, and the actions taken.
Essential documents	Documents which individually and collectively permit evaluation of the conduct of a study and the quality of the data produced.
Good Clinical Practice (GCP)	A standard for the design, conduct, performance monitoring, auditing, recording, analysis and reporting of clinical trials that provides assurance that the data and reported results are credible and accurate, and that the rights, integrity and confidentiality of trial subjects are protected.
Independent Data Monitoring Committee (IDMC) (also called the Data and Safety Monitoring Board)	An independent data-monitoring committee that may be established by the sponsor to assess at intervals the progress of a clinical trial, the safety data and the critical efficacy endpoints, and to recommend to the sponsor whether to continue, modify or stop a trial.
Impartial witness	A person, who is independent of the trial, who cannot be unfairly influenced by people involved with the trial, who attends the informed consent process if the subject or the subject's legally acceptable representative cannot read, and who reads the informed consent form and any other written information supplied to the subject.
Independent Ethics Committee (IEC)	An independent body (a review board or a committee, institutional, regional, national or supranational), constituted of medical professionals and nonmedical members, whose responsibility it is to ensure the protection of the rights, safety and well-being of human subjects involved in a trial and to provide public assurance of that protection by, among other things, reviewing and approving/providing favourable opinion on the trial protocol, the suitability of the investigator(s), facilities, and the methods and material to be used in obtaining and documenting informed consent of the trial subjects.
	The legal status, composition, function, operations and regulatory requirements pertaining to IECs may differ among countries, but should allow the IEC to act in agreement with GCP as described in this guideline.

continued

Table 5.5 Glossary of terms used in the conduct of clinical trials (*cont.*)

Term	Definition
Informed consent	A process by which a subject voluntarily confirms his or her willingness to participate in a particular trial, after having been informed of all aspects of the trial that are relevant to the subject's decision to participate. Informed consent is documented by means of a written, signed and dated informed consent form.
Inspection	The act by a regulatory authority or authorities of conducting an official review of documents, facilities, records and any other resources that are deemed by the authority or authorities to be related to the clinical trial and that may be located at the site of the trial, at the sponsor's and/or contract research organisation's (CRO's) facilities, or at other establishments deemed appropriate by the regulatory authority or authorities.
Institution (medical)	Any public or private entity or agency or medical or dental facility where clinical trials are conducted.
Institutional Review Board (IRB)	An independent body constituted of medical, scientific and nonscientific members, whose responsibility is to ensure the protection of the rights, safety and well-being of human subjects involved in a trial by, among other things, reviewing, approving and providing continuing review of trial protocol and amendments and of the methods and material to be used in obtaining and documenting informed consent of the trial subjects.
Interim clinical trial/study report	A report of intermediate results and their evaluation based on the analyses performed during the course of a trial.
Investigational product	A pharmaceutical form of an active ingredient or placebo being tested or used as a reference in a clinical trial, including a product with a marketing authorisation when used or assembled (formulated or packaged) in a way different from the approved form, or when used for an unapproved indication, or when used to gain further information about an approved use.
Investigator	A person responsible for the conduct of the clinical trial at a trial site. If a trial is conducted by a team of individuals at a trial site, the investigator is the responsible leader of the team and may be called the principal investigator. (See also Sub-investigator.)
Investigator/institution	An expression meaning 'the investigator and/or institution, where required by the applicable regulatory requirement(s)'.
Investigator's Brochure	A compilation of the clinical and nonclinical data on the investigational product(s) which is relevant to the study of the investigational product(s) in human subjects.
Legally acceptable representative	An individual or juridical or other body authorised under applicable law to consent, on behalf of a prospective subject, to the subject's participation in the clinical trial.

continued

Table 5.5 Glossary of terms used in the conduct of clinical trials (cont.)

Term	Definition
Monitoring	The act of overseeing the progress of a clinical trial, and of ensuring that it is conducted, recorded and reported in accordance with the protocol, standard operating procedures (SOPs), Good Clinical Practice (GCP) and the applicable regulatory requirement(s).
Monitoring report	A written report from the monitor to the sponsor after each site visit and/or other trial-related communication according to the sponsor's SOPs.
Multicentre trial	A clinical trial conducted according to a single protocol but at more than one site, and therefore carried out by more than one investigator.
Nonclinical study	Biomedical studies not performed on human subjects.
Opinion (in relation to Independent Ethics Committee)	The judgement and/or advice provided by an Independent Ethics Committee (IEC).
Protocol	A document that describes the objective(s), design, methodology, statistical considerations and organisation of a trial. The protocol usually also gives the background and rationale for the trial, but these could be provided in other protocol-referenced documents. Throughout the GCP guideline, the term 'protocol' refers to the protocol and protocol amendments.
Protocol amendment	A written description of change(s) to, or formal clarification of, a protocol.
Quality assurance	All those planned and systematic actions that are established to ensure that the trial is performed and the data are generated, documented (recorded) and reported in compliance with Good Clinical Practice (GCP) and the applicable regulatory requirement(s).
Quality control	The operational techniques and activities undertaken within the quality assurance system to verify that the requirements for quality of the trial-related activities have been fulfilled.
Randomisation	The process of assigning trial subjects to treatment or control groups using an element of chance to determine assignments in order to reduce bias.
Regulatory authorities	Bodies having the power to regulate. In this GCP guideline, the expression 'regulatory authorities' includes the authorities that review submitted clinical data and those that conduct inspections. These bodies are sometimes referred to as competent authorities.
Serious adverse event (SAE) or serious adverse drug reaction (serious ADR)	Any untoward medical occurrence that at any dose results in death, is life-threatening, requires in-patient hospitalisation or prolongation of existing hospitalisation, results in persistent or significant disability/incapacity, or is a congenital anomaly/birth defect. (See Note for Guidance on Clinical safety data management: definitions and standards for expedited reporting.)

continued

Table 5.5 Glossary of terms used in the conduct of clinical trials (*cont.*)

Term	Definition
Source data	All information in original records and certified copies of original records of clinical findings, observations or other activities in a clincal trial necessary for the reconstruction and evaluation of the trial. Source data are contained in source documents (original records or certified copies).
Source documents	Original documents, data and records (e.g. hospital records, clinical and office charts, laboratory notes, memoranda, subjects' diaries or evaluation checklists, pharmacy dispensing records, recorded data from automated instruments, copies or transcriptions certified after verification as being accurate copies, microfiches, photographic negatives, microfilm or magnetic media, radiographs, subject files, and records kept at the pharmacy, at the laboratories and at medicotechnical departments involved in the clinical trial).
Sponsor	An individual, company, institution or organisation which takes responsibility for the initiation, management and/or financing of a clinical trial.
Sponsor-investigator	An individual who both initiates and conducts, alone or with others, a clinical trial and under whose immediate direction the investigational product is administered to, dispensed to or used by a subject. The term does not include any person other than an individual (e.g. it does not include a corporation or any agency). The obligations of a sponsor-investigator include both those of a sponsor and those of an investigator.
Standard operating procedures (SOPs)	Detailed written instructions to achieve uniformity of the performance of a specific function.
Sub-investigator	Any individual member of the clinical trial team designated and supervised by the investigator at a trial site to perform critical trial-related procedures and/or to make important trial-related decisions (e.g. associates, residents, research fellows). (See also Investigator.)
Subject/trial subject	An individual who participates in a clinical trial, either as a recipient of the investigational product(s) or as a control.
Subject identification code	A unique identifier assigned by the investigator to each trial subject to protect the subject's identity and used in lieu of the subject's name when the investigator reports adverse events and/or trial-related data.
Trial site	The location(s) where trial-related activities are actually conducted.
Unexpected adverse drug reaction	An adverse reaction, the nature or severity of which is not consistent with the applicable product information (e.g. Investigator's Brochure for an unapproved investigational product or package, or Summary of Product Characteristics for an approved product) (see Note for Guidance on Clinical safety data management: definitions and standards for expedited reporting).

continued

Table 5.5 Glossary of terms used in the conduct of clinical trials (*cont.*)

Term	Definition
Vulnerable subjects	Individuals whose willingness to volunteer in a clinical trial may be unduly influenced by the expectation, whether justified or not, of benefits associated with participation, or of a retaliatory response from senior members of a hierarchy in case of refusal to participate. Examples are members of a group with a hierarchical structure such as medical, pharmacy, dental and nursing students, subordinate hospital and laboratory personnel, employees of the pharmaceutical industry, members of the armed forces and persons kept in detention. Other vulnerable subjects include patients with incurable diseases, persons in nursing homes, unemployed or impoverished persons, patients in emergency situations, ethnic minority groups, homeless persons, nomads, refugees, minors and those incapable of giving consent.
Well-being (of the trial subjects)	The physical and mental integrity of the subjects participating in a clinical trial.

Equally importantly, the investigational products must be manufactured, handled and stored in accordance with current Good Manufacturing Practice (GMP) and in accordance with the written protocol.

Independent Ethics Committees

The IEC exists to protect the well-being of subjects recruited into clinical trials, and to ensure that the protocol is adequate and professional. In order to assess this, the IEC expects to study the following documents:

- trial protocol (and any amendments)
- written informed consent forms
- subject recruitment procedures
- written information provided to potential subjects
- the Investigator's Brochure
- available safety information
- information about payments and compensation available to participants
- the investigator's CV and proof of qualifications.

On-going trials are reviewed by the IEC at intervals dependent upon the risk to subjects in the trial, but at least once a year.

The IEC has to determine whether the protocol for a trial with a nontherapeutic agent carried out with the consent of the subject's legally acceptable representative satisfies ethical concerns and relevant regulatory requirements. The IEC also has to safeguard the well-being of a trial subject when prior consent to participate in the trial cannot be given.

Payments

Payment for participation in a trial is a potentially problematic issue, and the IEC must ensure that the amount and method of any payment agreed with participants is acceptable and reasonable. The payment also needs to be divided such that receiving the expected fee is not entirely dependent upon completion of the trial by the subject.

Membership of the IEC

There must be a range of expertise present within the membership of the IEC that provides the ability to assess the scientific, medical and ethical aspects of a trial. There should be at least five members, one of whom should have a primary interest in a nonscientific specialty, and one of whom must be independent of the trial site and organisation.

Operating procedures

Organised and run like any well-constituted committee, the IEC must have written operating procedures, keep written minutes of meetings and decisions, and comply with GCP and relevant regulatory requirements. A quorum must be present for any decisions taken, and only those who have been present and participated in the deliberations of the IEC can vote on any issues.

Written operating procedures should include details of the scheduling of meetings and conducting and timing of trial reviews. The IEC must also determine that no modifications should be made to the trial protocol without its approval, other than when necessary to eliminate immediate dangers to the trial subjects or to make minor logistical changes (e.g. an amendment to a telephone number). The IEC also defines what issues the investigator needs to report: these may include all adverse drug reactions (ADRs) and changes that need to be made to the conduct of the trial.

Records

All relevant records must be kept by the IEC for at least 3 years after the completion of the trial. The documentation must also be available to be reviewed by the regulatory authority or authorities.

Investigator

The investigator must be adequately and appropriately qualified to be in charge of the trial and be able to provide documentation to the sponsor, the IEC and the regulatory authority that supports this. He or she must also be thoroughly familiar with all aspects of the actions and effects of the investigational product being used in the trial. An awareness of GCP, and an ability to enforce it, is necessary; this includes allowing monitoring and auditing of the trial to take place.

Resources

The resources available to the investigator must allow the investigator to demonstrate that he or she can recruit sufficient subjects into the trial within the agreed time, and that there is adequate time allowed for the effective conduct of the trial. A full range of support staff must be available, each of whom is fully trained and briefed on the protocol, the investigational product and their duties.

Medical care of the subjects

It is necessary for a qualified physician to be an investigator or subinvestigator for the trial who can take all the trial-related medical decisions. There must also be adequate medical facilities to be able to deal with any adverse events. It is also normally expected that the trial physician will notify the subject's physician about their participation in the trial (if the subject agrees and has a primary physician).

The investigator is responsible for regular communications with the IEC and for informing the IEC of any untoward changes in the conduct of the trial. He or she is also responsible for ensuring that there is compliance with the approved protocol and for not permitting any deviations from it unless there is an urgent clinical need to do so and the changes are approved retrospectively by the IEC.

Investigational product

In theory, the investigator is also responsible for the investigational product and its accountability throughout the trial. In practice, this is usually delegated to a trial pharmacist. The pharmacist should keep records of the delivery of the product to the trial site, the stocks held at the site, the usage by each subject and the return to the sponsor of any unused product. Safe and secure storage of the product is essential. The investigator, usually through the trial pharmacist, is also aware of the degree of randomisation of the trial and the procedures for 'unblinding' of the trial (e.g. in the event of an adverse event or accidental revelation of the randomisation process).

Informed consent

All ethical guidelines (e.g. appropriate regulatory guidelines and the Declaration of Helsinki) must be followed in obtaining a subject's informed consent. There must be written procedures for a subject to give consent which have been approved by the IEC. There must also not be undue coercion for a subject to participate in a trial.

Full information about the trial, and the approval given for it by the IEC, must be communicated to the subject prior to their giving consent. This information should be presented in nontechnical language, and any questions that the subject may have must be answered fully. If the subject cannot give informed consent personally (e.g. owing to their medical condition or age), a legally acceptable representative can do so, accompanied by an impartial witness to the signing of the consent form if the legally acceptable representative cannot read the form.

Information that must be provided to a subject giving informed consent includes:

- that the trial involves research
- the purpose of the trial and how a subject will be assigned to a group during the trial
- those aspects of the trial that are experimental
- those risks and benefits that can be reasonably foreseen in participating in the trial
- compensation or treatment available should there arise a trial-related injury
- payments (and their interval) and expenses to be paid
- confirmation that the participation in the trial is voluntary
- recognition that the monitor, auditors, IEC and the regulatory authority will be given access to the subject's original medical records without violating their confidentiality
- the expected duration of the trial.

In an emergency situation, where it is not possible to obtain the prior consent of the subject, that of the legally acceptable representative can be sought. When neither of these options is available, the subject can be enrolled in the trial following procedures laid down in the protocol that have been agreed by the IEC. In all cases, the safety and well-being of the subject are paramount and there must be compliance with all regulatory requirements. Consent should be sought from either the subject or their legally acceptable representative at the earliest subsequent opportunity.

Records and reports

Data are reported to the sponsor by the investigator using case report forms (CRFs), whose content must be consistent with the source documents. CRFs are retained for future reference and measures are taken to prevent their accidental destruction. They must be retained for at least 2 years after the last approval of an MAA or at least 2 years after completion of clinical development of the investigational product. (They may need to be held for longer under the requirements of some regulatory authorities.) All reports and records must be held available for inspection by the monitor, auditor, IEC and regulatory authority.

Safety reporting

The investigator must report all serious adverse events to the sponsor immediately, and follow up a verbal report with a written report. Adverse events must be reported using the unique code number assigned to a subject, maintaining confidentiality. In the event of death of a subject, further information (e.g. autopsy reports) must also be forwarded by the investigator.

Premature termination or suspension of a trial

If a trial is terminated, the investigator must notify the trial subjects and ensure that their continued medical treatment is appropriate; the investigator must also inform the regulatory authorities concerned. Whether it is the investigator or sponsor who stops the trial, a detailed explanation must be given to the IEC.

Sponsor

Quality assurance and quality control

Written standard operating proceedures (SOPs) are required that trials are conducted in compliance with the protocol, GCP and appropriate regulatory requirements. Similar constraints apply to the data generated, documented and recorded. Monitoring and auditing by the sponsor must be carried out at trial sites, and all documentation must be made directly available to the sponsor. All interested parties must also allow inspections by their national and foreign regulatory authorities.

Contract research organisation

Companies may delegate, under written agreements, some or all trial-related activities to a contract research organisation. Nevertheless, the ultimate responsibility for the trial and its conduct lies with the sponsor.

Medical expertise

Appropriately qualified medical personnel, either employed directly by the sponsor or on a consultancy basis, must be made available by the sponsor to advise on trial-related medical problems.

Trial design

The design of the trial, its conduct and the protocol must be prepared under the guidance of the sponsor by appropriately qualified staff.

Trial management, data handling and record-keeping

The conduct of the trial, and the preparation, verification and statistical analysis of the data must be carried out by appropriately qualified staff. An independent data-monitoring committee may assess the trial's progress and offer advice to the sponsor on whether a trial should continue.

Trial data are increasingly being developed electronically, for which appropriate written safeguards and protocols must be generated. An audit trail must be achieved, especially to identify changes to the data, and there must be an adequate security system that controls and monitors personnel making changes.

If the sponsor discontinues a trial, all relevant documentation must be retained for at least 2 years after termination, and the sponsor must notify the appropriate regulatory authorities of the decision. Documentation must also be retained for at least 2 years after the last approval of a marketing authorisation in an ICH region, or until there are no pending or contemplated MAAs in an ICH region.

Investigator selection

Suitably qualified and trained investigators are selected by the sponsor under a written agreement. The investigator must agree to conduct the trial according to GCP and the relevant regulatory requirements and using the written protocol approved by the sponsor and the IEC. There must be compliance with record-keeping requirements, and the investigator must permit monitoring, auditing and inspection.

Compensation to subjects and investigators

Insurance or indemnity should be provided by the sponsor against potential claims arising from the trial or related activities. Any compensation payments must be made in accordance with regulatory requirements.

Notification to regulatory authorities

The sponsor is responsible for submitting any required applications to regulatory authorities prior to the trial starting.

Confirmation of review by the IEC

The investigator must supply to the sponsor his or her name and address, written confirmation that operations are carried out according to GCP standards, and written proof of approval having been obtained from the IEC.

Manufacturing and packaging of the investigational product

All investigational products used in the trial must be manufactured to GMP standards and coded to protect the blinding of the trial. Transport and storage conditions may need to be carefully controlled to prevent product deterioration, depending upon its physical characteristics. Should a medical emergency warrant it, the coding should be organised to allow rapid identification of the product's identity by an authorised person.

Supplying and handling the investigational product

It is the sponsor's responsibility to supply the investigators with the trial product once all the preliminary documentation has been satisfactorily completed. Full details of the optimal transport and storage conditions must be explained by the sponsor to the investigator. All shipments must be fully documented and that documentation retained as one of the trial's essential documents.

Access to records

The investigator must allow the sponsor direct access to the all documents needed for monitoring the trial, auditing, review by the IEC and regulatory inspection.

Adverse drug reaction reporting

Serious and unexpected ADRs must be notified by the sponsor to the investigator, to the IEC and, where required, to the regulatory authority. Safety updates and periodic reports may also need to be submitted by the sponsor to the regulatory authority.

Monitoring

Monitoring helps ensure that the rights and well-being of trial subjects are protected, that the data generated in the trial are valid and accurate, and that the trial is being conducted according to GCP requirements.

Monitors must be appropriately qualified and be made fully aware of all aspects of the investigational product and the conduct of the trial. They are appointed by the sponsor in numbers that reflect the complexity and size of the trial and its endpoints. Monitors in effect act as liaison channels between the investigator and the sponsor and ensure that the trial is carried out according to the sponsor's written instructions. The range of their functions may vary between trials, but in essence they are responsible for verifying:

- that the investigator's qualifications and resources are adequate throughout the trial
- that the trial product is stored and handled appropriately
- compliance with the protocol
- that informed consent has been obtained from all subjects
- that the investigator has all documentation needed to carry out the trial in compliance with regulatory requirements
- that only eligible subjects are recruited into the trial and that sufficient numbers are available for the trial
- the accuracy and completeness of the case report forms for each subject
- that all ADR reports and adverse event reports are fully documented
- that all essential documentation is completed.

Monitors have to prepare a written report for the sponsor after each trial site visit that outlines the significant facts and findings from the visit, any deficiencies and deviations from the protocol identified, and any action that is required for the investigator to carry out.

Audit

The process of audit carried out for the sponsor is independent of the trial's quality control procedures. The primary purpose of an audit is to evaluate the conduct of the trial and to ensure compliance with the protocol and all other written and regulatory procedures.

It is the sponsor's responsibility to detail what is to be audited, how the audit is to be carried out and how frequently, and the structure and content of the audit report. These issues will be determined by the complexity of the trial, its size and the potential risk to participants. Unless there is a problem of noncompliance with GCP or legal proceedings require their release, it is usual for regulatory authorities not to regularly request to see audit reports. This helps to maintain the independence and value of the audit function.

Noncompliance

A sponsor must take prompt action to redress failure to comply with the protocol, SOPs, GCP and regulatory requirements by the investigator and/or institution. Should this noncompliance be persistent, the involvement of those guilty must be terminated by the sponsor, and this action reported to the regulatory authority.

Premature suspension or termination of a trial

If, for whatever reason, a trial is suspended or terminated, the sponsor must notify those involved: the institution, the investigator, the regulatory authority and the IEC. It is still necessary for the sponsor to supply to the regulatory authority all the clinical trial reports.

Multicentre trials

A sponsor of any trial that is carried out in a number of different locations, which may be spread over several countries or continents, has to ensure that all locations comply with all of the above requirements.

Clinical trial protocol and protocol amendments

The trial protocol is a crucial document outlining all aspects of the trial and its performance. If any information is contained in other trial documents, these further documents must be cross-referenced to the trial protocol. The core information must include the following:

- general information
- background information

- trial objectives and purpose
- trial design
- selection and withdrawal of subjects
- treatment of subjects
- assessment of efficacy
- assessment of safety
- statistics
- direct access to source data/documents
- quality control and quality assurance
- ethics
- data handling and record keeping
- financing and insurance
- publication policy
- supplements.

More detailed information on the data required under each heading is given in Table 5.6.

Table 5.6 Clinical trial protocol requirements

General information
- Protocol title, identifying number and date. Any amendments should also bear the amendment number and date
- Name and address of sponsor and monitor
- Name and title of the person(s) authorised to sign the protocol and any amendments for the sponsor
- Name, title, address and telephone number of the sponsor's medical expert for the trial
- Name and title of the investigator(s) who is/are responsible for conducting the trial, and the address and telephone number(s) of the trial site(s)
- Name, title, address and telephone number of the qualified physician responsible for all trial-related medical decisions
- Name and address of the clinical laboratory and other medical and/or technical departments/institutions involved in the trial

Background information
- Name and description of the investigational product
- Summary of findings from nonclinical studies that potentially have clinical significance and from clinical trials that are relevant to the trial
- Summary of known and potential risks and benefits, if any, to human subjects
- Description of and justification for the route of administration, dosage, dosage regimen and treatment periods
- A statement that the trial will be conducted in compliance with the protocol, GCP and applicable regulatory requirements
- Description of the population to be studied
- References to literature and data that are relevant to the trial and that provide background for the trial

Trial objectives and purpose
- A detailed description of the objectives and purpose of the trial

Trial design
- A specific statement of the primary and secondary endpoints to be measured
- A description of the type and design of the trial (e.g. double-blind, placebo-controlled, parallel design) and a schematic diagram of trial design, procedure and stages
- A description of the measures to be taken to minimise/avoid bias, including randomisation and blinding
- The trial treatment and the dosage and dosage regimen of the investigational product. A description of the dosage form, the packaging and the labelling of the investigational product should also be given
- The expected duration of subject participation and a description of the sequence and duration of all trial periods, including any follow-up

continued

Table 5.6 Clinical trial protocol requirements (*cont.*)

- A description of the 'stopping rules' or 'discontinuation criteria' of individual subjects, parts of the trial and the entire trial
- Accountability procedures for the investigational product, including the placebo and comparator (if any)
- Maintenance of the trial randomisation codes and procedures for breaking codes
- The identification of any data to be recorded directly on the Case Report Forms and to be considered to be source data

Selection and withdrawal of subjects
- Subject inclusion and exclusion criteria
- Subject withdrawal criteria and procedures specifying when and how to withdraw subjects from the trial, the type and timing of the data to be collected for withdrawn subjects, whether and how subjects are to be replaced, and the follow-up for subjects withdrawn from the trial

Treatment of subjects
- The treatment to be administered, including:
  name of the product
  dose
  dosing schedule
  route and mode of administration
  treatment period, including the follow-up period
- Medication and treatment allowed (including rescue medication) and not allowed before and during the trial
- Procedures for monitoring compliance

Assessment of efficacy
- Specification of efficacy parameters
- Methods and timing for assessing, recording and analysing efficacy parameters

Assessment of safety
- Specification of safety parameters
- Methods and timing for assessing, recording and analysing safety parameters
- Procedures for eliciting reports of, and recording and reporting, adverse events and intercurrent illnesses
- The type and duration of the follow-up of subjects after adverse events

Statistics
- A description of the statistical methods to be used, including timing of any planned interim analyses
- The number of subjects planned to be enrolled. In multicentre trials, the number of enrolled subjects projected for each trial site should be specified. Reason for choice of sample size, including reflections on (or calculations of) the power of the trial and clinical justification
- The level of significance to be used
- Criteria for termination of the trial
- Procedure for accounting for missing, unused and spurious data
- Procedures for reporting any deviations from the original statistical plan
- The selection of subjects to be included in the analyses (e.g. all randomised subjects, all dosed subjects, all eligible subjects, evaluable subjects)

Direct access to source data/documents
- The sponsor should ensure that it is specified in the protocol or other written agreement that the investigator will permit trial-related monitoring, audits, IEC review, and regulatory inspection, providing direct access to source data and documents

Quality control and quality assurance
Ethics
- Description of ethical considerations relating to the trial

Data handling and record keeping
Financing and insurance
- If not addressed in a separate agreement

Publication policy
- If not addressed in a separate agreement

Supplements

Investigator's Brochure

The Investigator's Brochure comprises a summary of the clinical and nonclinical data on the investigational product for the clinical trial and is provided to the investigators, who are subsequently responsible for it being sent to the IEC. In essence, it explains why the trial is taking place and why various critical aspects of the trial (e.g. dose, methods of administration and safety monitoring procedures) have been selected. The brochure also details how the subjects enrolled in the trial should be managed clinically. When prepared in a simple and nonpromotional way, it allows the investigating clinician to assess the potential risk/benefit of the trial.

The amount of information provided in the Investigator's Brochure will vary depending upon the stage of the development of the trial product. For a previously marketed and well-established product, there is usually need only for a brochure of limited scope. The brochure should also be updated at least once a year, or more frequently if new relevant information is determined prior to annual updating.

Examples of a title page and a table of contents of an Investigator's Brochure are given in Table 5.7.

The content of most sections of the Investigator's Brochure is self-explanatory. The Summary should preferably not exceed two pages, but should cover all information available at the particular stage of development. The Introduction should give the names of the product (chemical, generic and trade name), its pharmacological class and potential advantages of the new product over existing therapies, why the research is being conducted and the product's likely indications.

Details of the formulation, including excipients, are necessary to permit action in the event of a safety problem. Appropriate storage and handling guidelines should also be provided.

Studies carried out on nonclinical pharmacology, toxicology, pharmacokinetics and metabolism should be summarised. Data should include the species tested, dose interval and duration, and the findings evaluated.

Human studies already carried out should be explained and information should be included on pharmacodynamics, dose response, safety and efficacy. Countries in which the investigational product has already been marketed should be listed, and any relevant findings from previous marketing explained.

Clinical trials Directive (Directive 2001/20/EC)

Despite being one of the most important elements of the data required for the submission of an MAA, until recently there was no pan-European legislation which governed the conduct of clinical trials. Such legislation as

Table 5.7 Investigator's Brochure – sample title page and table of contents

Title page (example)
Sponsor's name:
Product:
Research number:
Name: chemical, generic (if approved)
　　　　trade name(s) (if legally permissible and desired by the sponsor)

Investigator's Brochure
Edition number:
Release date:
Replaces previous edition number:
Date:

Table of contents (example)
Confidentiality statement (optional)
Signature page (optional)

1. Table of contents
2. Summary
3. Introduction
4. Physical, chemical and pharmaceutical properties and formulation
5. Nonclinical studies
　　5.1　Nonclinical pharmacology
　　5.2　Pharmacokinetics and product metabolism in animals
　　5.3　Toxicology
6. Effects in humans
　　6.1　Pharmacokinetics and product metabolism in humans
　　6.2　Safety and efficacy
　　6.3　Marketing experience
7. Summary of data and guidance for the investigator

References (literature references to publications and reports should be located at the end of each chapter)
Appendices (if any)

---

existed was national legislation, as a consequence of which there were significant differences in the requirements within each EU Member State as to how clinical trials should be undertaken and controlled.

The concept of GCP applied to clinical trials is described above. However, GCP cannot be enforced by legislation as its implementation in clinical trials is subject only to a guideline, not a Directive or Regulation. Directive 2001/20/EC therefore represents the first time that statutory controls have been put in place to define the ways in which clinical trials are carried out.

Reasons for the legislation

The primary EU legislation for the control of the authorisation of human medicinal products is the Community Code (Directive 2001/83/EC). This Directive rationalised and standardised all pre-existing European legislation relating to human medicinal products that had been passed since the first such Directive 65/65/EEC in 1965. The Code requires that MAAs should be accompanied by data containing the particulars and documents relating to the results of clinical trials carried out on a medicinal product. Part 4 of Annex I to Directive 2001/83/EC gives guidance on the documentation on clinical trials which must be submitted, and also includes a requirement that all phases of clinical investigation should be designed, implemented and reported in accordance with the principles of GCP.

As a result of the significant differences that have developed over the years in the national requirements for carrying out clinical trials across the EU, legislation has been introduced in an attempt to simplify and harmonise the administration of clinical trials. Directive 2001/20/EC establishes a clear and transparent procedure that is intended to allow more effective co-ordination of trials within the EU by the regulatory authorities.

Although the administrative processes are intended to be harmonised by the introduction of the new Directive, it was recognised at the outset of its drafting that there would remain significant differences in the way that clinical trials are actually conducted in each EU Member State. Had it been intended to entirely harmonise clinical trial practices across the EU, the European Commission would have had to introduce a Regulation, which would automatically have been applicable in all Member States. Instead, a decision was made to introduce a Directive, which has to be transposed into national legislation in each country. The new Directive should harmonise the administrative processes, but the underlying practice and conduct of clinical trials will continue to vary across the EU.

Objectives and major changes introduced

The full title of the legislation – Directive 2001/20/EC relating to the implementation of good clinical practice in the conduct of clinical trials on medicinal products for human use – explains its primary purpose. After considerable negotiation and consultation within the European Commission, agreement on the finalised version of the Directive was reached in February 2001, which was then published on 1 May 2001. An implementation period of 3 years for the legislation was set; hence its provisions had to enter into force in each EU Member State by 1 May 2004.

Implementation in the UK

The legislation was implemented in the UK by the Medicines for Human Use (Clinical Trials) Regulations 2003. National implementation significantly changed the way in which clinical trials within the UK were controlled. Under the former UK system, control was directed towards the supply of a medicinal product for a clinical trial. Under the new system, the procedures which must be undertaken to start and carry out a clinical trial and the manufacturing process of any medicinal product(s) used in the trial (referred to as 'investigational medicinal products', IMPs) are controlled and monitored.

In addition, previously the person wishing to supply a medicinal product for a clinical trial in the UK had to obtain a Clinical Trial Certificate (CTC) or a Clinical Trial Exemption certificate (CTX). Now it is necessary to obtain a clinical trial authorisation from the regulatory authority. The new controls also placed on a legal basis the ethics committee approval that must be obtained prior to starting a trial, and which resulted in the creation of a new UK Ethics Committee Authority.

Protection of subjects

One of the other major objectives of the Directive is that it sets out standards for the protection of subjects enrolled in clinical trials, and in particular incapacitated adults and minors. In effect, the Directive is intended to protect participants in trials by the introduction of GCP principles into the regulation and conduct of clinical trials.

Main points of the Directive

Directive 2001/20/EC has a particularly wide scope and applies to every clinical trial on medicinal products, whether sponsored by the pharmaceutical industry, by government, by research organisations or by a charity or a university. It emphasises that the basis for the conduct of clinical trials is the protection of human rights and the dignity of human beings, as reflected in the Declaration of Helsinki. Prior to a clinical trial being carried out, the potential risk to participants must have been assessed by carrying out animal toxicological experiments, by screening undertaken by ethics committees and the drug regulatory authority, and by compliance with the rules on the protection of personal data.

Clinical trials in children

The situation of clinical trials conducted in children is more complicated. It is essential that trials to develop medicinal products for children are undertaken whenever possible, but with the clear recognition that children represent a vulnerable population. They are at a different stage of development and have different physiological and psychological characteristics from adults. As a result, their response to the administration of particular medicinal products will inevitably be different from that of an adult. One of the most important classes of medicine available for children, and in which clinical trials are essential prior to their use, is that of vaccines used against childhood diseases. The Directive lays down the criteria for the protection of children in clinical trials.

Problems in giving informed consent

The Directive emphasises the need for those who are incapable of giving informed consent to their participation in a trial to be given special protection. Moreover, no such person can be included in a trial if the same results could be obtained using a person who can give their informed consent to their participation. Those unable to give their informed consent should only be included when it is likely that the administration of the drug would be of direct benefit to them as individuals.

For adults who are unable to give their informed consent (e.g. those suffering from dementia or those who are psychiatric patients), the Directive imposes even stricter controls. As with trials in children, there must be seen to be a clear potential benefit for the individual participating in the trial. In addition, if their inclusion is deemed to be essential, the written consent of the patient's legal representative must be obtained prior to starting any trial, and must be obtained in co-operation with the treating doctor.

As one of the primary objectives of the legislation is to provide protection for participants in clinical trials, the Directive also requires that obsolete or repetitive tests should not be carried out at any time. The legislation recognises that the harmonisation of the technical requirements for the registration of medicinal products under the ICH process will help to reduce the likelihood of repetitive tests being carried out in different global regions.

Administrative procedures

A new European database is to be established in which information on the content, start dates and finishing dates of a clinical trial is to be recorded. The data are to be made available to the regulatory authorities in Member States in which the trial is taking place and to all other Member State regulatory authorities.

As mentioned above, there are currently significant differences in the ways in which Member States carry out the control and conduct of clinical trials in their own territories. This has led to delays and complications, preventing the effective conduct of clinical trials throughout Europe. The administrative provisions for clinical trials are therefore being harmonised and simplified in order to create a clear and transparent procedure across the EU, thereby enhancing the co-ordination of authorisation of trials by the regulatory authorities.

In theory, the application to begin a clinical trial submitted to an ethics committee and to a regulatory authority should be deemed to be approved unless a definite negative response has been received from one of those two bodies. Only if there has been significant interaction between the approving bodies and the applicant on various aspects of the clinical trial application would a formal, explicit authorisation be deemed to be necessary.

Investigational medicinal products

Investigational medicinal products should be prepared in accordance with the principles of good manufacturing practice (GMP) with appropriate labelling of such products.

The Directive recognises that noncommercial clinical trials frequently take place without the participation of the pharmaceutical industry and therefore without their considerable resources to underpin the trial activities. Such trials usually take place with medicinal products that are already authorised and which are therefore manufactured in accordance with the principles of GMP. The trials are usually undertaken to further investigate the indications already approved for a particular medicinal product. It is proposed within the Directive that there should be simplified labelling of investigational medicinal products laid down in the GMP guidelines.

Conformity with GCP

All clinical trials must be undertaken to the standards of GCP, with the corresponding need for the data collected during the trial to be properly recorded and reported in order to justify the involvement of human subjects in the trial. Moreover, any individual participating in a clinical trial must give informed consent to the scrutiny of personal data by the regulatory authority and by the ethics committee, and be reassured that the data are treated in a strictly confidential manner.

Scope of the Directive

The Directive includes for the first time not only clinical trials on patients who are intended to benefit from the course of treatment administered but also those involving healthy volunteers (Phase I trials). In effect, all trials that are undertaken with a medicinal product are subject to the terms of the Directive, which includes both commercial and noncommercial research. This is a major change for the UK, although in implementing the requirement the UK has been brought more into line with the current situation in almost all other EU Member States.

A number of definitions are given in the Directive (see Table 5.8). Several issues arise from the definitions given.

A 'clinical trial' is any activity in which the safety and efficacy of a medicinal product is being assessed. Under these circumstances, a clinical trial authorisation is required. For any product that is used in a clinical trial, either as a test product or as a reference product, a manufacturing authorisation is also required.

Table 5.8 Definitions: Directive 2001/20/EC

Term	Definition
Clinical trial	Any investigation in human subjects intended to discover or verify the clinical, pharmacological and/or pharmacodynamic effects of one or more investigational medicinal product(s), and/or to identify any adverse reactions to one or more investigational medicinal product(s), and/or to study absorption, distribution, metabolism and excretion of one or more investigational medicinal product(s) with the object of assessing its (their) safety and/or efficacy. This includes clinical trials carried out in either one site or multiple sites, whether in one or more than one Member State.
Multicentre clinical trial	A clinical trial conducted according to a single protocol but at more than one site, and therefore by more than one investigator, in which the trial sites may be located in a single Member State, in a number of Member States, and/or in Member States and third countries.
Noninterventional trial	A study where the medicinal product(s) is(are) prescribed in the usual manner in accordance with the terms of the marketing authorisation. The assignment of the patient to a particular therapeutic strategy is not decided in advance by a trial protocol but falls within current practice and the prescription of the medicine is clearly separated from the decision to include the patient in the study. No additional diagnostic or monitoring procedures shall be applied to the patients and epidemiological methods shall be used the analysis of collected data.
Investigational medicinal product	A pharmaceutical form of an active substance or placebo being tested or used as a reference in a clinical trial, including products already with a marketing authorisation but used or assembled (formulated or packaged) in a way different from the authorised form, or when used for an unauthorised indication, or when used to gain further information about the authorised form.
Sponsor	An individual, company, institution or organisation which takes responsibility for the initiation, management and/or financing of a clinical trial.
Investigator	A doctor or person following a profession agreed in the Member State for investigations because of their scientific background and the experience in patient care it requires. The investigator is responsible for the conduct of a clinical trial at a trial site. If a trial is conducted by a team of individuals at a trial site, the investigator is the leader responsible for the team and may be called the principal investigator.
Investigator's Brochure	A compilation of the clinical and nonclinical data on the investigational medicinal product or products which are relevant to the study of the product or products in human subjects.
Protocol	A document that describes the objective(s), design, methodology, statistical considerations and organisation of a trial. The term 'protocol' refers to the protocol, successive versions of the protocol and protocol amendments.
Subject	An individual who participates in a clinical trial as either a recipient of the investigational medicinal product or a control.

continued

Table 5.8 Definitions: Directive 2001/20/EC (*cont.*)

Term	Definition
Informed consent	A decision, which must be written, dated and signed, to take part in a clinical trial, taken freely after being duly informed of its nature, significance, implications and risks, and appropriately documented, by any person capable of giving consent or, where the person is not capable of giving consent, by his or her legal representative. If the person is unable to write, oral consent in the presence of at least one witness may be given in exceptional cases, as provided for in national legislation.
Ethics committee	An independent body in a Member State, consisting of healthcare professionals and nonmedical members, whose responsibility it is to protect the rights, safety and well-being of human subjects involved in a trial and to provide public assurance of that protection by, among other things, expressing an opinion on the trial protocol, the suitability of the investigators and the adequacy of facilities, and on the methods and documents to be used to inform trial subjects and obtain their informed consent.
Inspection	The act by a competent authority of conducting an official review of documents, facilities, records, quality assurance arrangements and any other resources that are deemed by the competent authority to be related to the clinical trial and that may be located at the site of the trial, at the sponsor's and/or contract research organisation's facilities, or at other establishments which the competent authority sees fit to inspect.
Adverse event	Any untoward medical occurrence in a patient or clinical trial subject administered a medicinal product and which does not necessarily have a causal relationship with this treatment.
Adverse reaction	All untoward and unintended responses to an investigatinal medicinal product related to any dose administered.
Serious adverse event or serious adverse reaction	Any untoward medical occurrence or effect that at any dose results in death, is life-threatening, requires hospitalisation or prolongation of existing hospitalisation, results in persistent or significant disability or incapacity, or is a congenital anomaly or birth defect.
Unexpected adverse reaction	An adverse reaction, the nature or severity of which is not consistent with the applicable product information (e.g. Investigator's Brochure for an unauthorised investigational medicinal product or Summary of Product Characteristics for an authorised product).

'Noninterventional trials' are excluded from the definition of a clinical trial. In such trials a medicinal product is usually administered in a way which falls within current practice and there is no separation of patients into reference or placebo groups prior to administration. Moreover, no additional diagnostic or monitoring procedures are applied to the patients. In other words, patient are receiving the same treatment as they would under normal clinical care. Should this remain the case, the study is classed as 'noninterventional.'

A 'sponsor' is any entity which takes responsibility for starting, managing and/or financing a clinical trial. In the UK, many clinical trials, and especially Phase I studies, have been carried out in collaboration between universities, the NHS and research councils and/or charities. In such cases, the sponsor would be the individual body which takes on this ultimate responsibility for the trial. It is necessary for those involved in the conduct of the trial to determine and to agree upon who is the sponsor for a particular trial and for that nominee to be notified to the regulatory authorities.

Protection of clinical trial subjects

It is essential that a clinical trial is only undertaken when there is considered to be a possible benefit for the individual taking part in the trial, and for future patients. The anticipated therapeutic and public health benefits should justify the risks, and the assessment of this criterion is carried by an ethics committee and by the regulatory authority. The clinical trial is also permanently monitored to ensure that the continued benefits justify the risks.

It is essential that the participants in the trial have been fully informed of its objectives, the risks entailed and possible inconvenience in their participation. Participants must also have been advised of their right to withdraw from the trial at any time without prejudice. If the participants are unable to give informed consent, the same explanation should be given to their legal representatives. If a participant is not able to physically write their informed consent, oral consent may be obtained as long as it is in the presence of at least one witness, whose role should then be recorded.

The investigator and sponsor should ensure that insurance or indemnity has been obtained to cover their liabilities for the clinical trial. It is also essential that the care of the subjects taking part in the trial is maintained under an appropriately qualified medical doctor.

Clinical trials on minors

The legislation recognises the difficulties in obtaining informed consent from a minor, drawing particular attention to the capacity of understanding displayed by the individual about what is being proposed by their participation in the clinical trial. If the young person understands what is being proposed but refuses to participate or requests to be withdrawn from the clinical trial at any time, this decision must be respected. Moreover, no incentives or financial inducements should be given to the child other than compensation.

One of the other important aspects of the legislation is that there should be some direct benefit for the group of patients, and that the trial should only be carried out when its essential to validate data obtained in clinical trials where participants have been able to give their informed consent. In addition, the clinical trial and its objectives should relate directly to the condition from which the young person is suffering, or it must be such that the trial can only be carried out on this particular age group.

Clinical trials in all age groups should be undertaken and designed so as to minimise the level of pain, discomfort, fear and other risks. These requirements are especially important when it comes to undertaking clinical trials in children and young people.

Those unable to give informed legal consent

The inability to be able to give informed consent to participation in a clinical trial can often arise because of serious or life-threatening conditions, or because the ability of the individual to understand what is being requested is severely restricted. Whenever possible, as much information as is likely to be understood should be given to an incapacitated adult. Again, as with young patients, should there be any indication that the individual does not want to participate in the trial, this should be respected.

The informed consent of the incapacitated adult's legal representative must be obtained in place of that of the participant. The consent given by the legal representative must represent what the individual would presumably have decided had they been able to make the choice for themselves.

As in the case of clinical trials on minors, it is vital that the interests of the patient always prevail over those of science and society in general. The role of the ethics committee in assessing the involvement of an incapacitated adult is vital in ensuring that the rights and interests of the individual are always respected and maintained.

The legal representative may be someone classed as a 'personal legal representative' who is chosen as a consequence of the relationship with the potential participant in the clinical trial. This might be a member of the close or extended family or someone who can demonstrate a close personal relationship with the individual concerned. By comparison, if no-one appropriate can be identified for that purpose, a 'professional legal representative' should act for the individual.

In some cases, the issue of potential participation in a clinical trial may arise at very short notice (e.g. after cardiac arrest or following a severe head injury). It can often be difficult to locate an appropriate person to act as a personal legal representative. The likelihood of this situation arising would previously have been identified in the protocol submitted to an ethics committee, and the procedure to be followed would have been approved by the ethics committee prior to starting the clinical trial. The Directive does not seek to prevent emergency research being carried out.

Ethics committees

For the first time, the role of an ethics committee has been brought under statutory provisions. The function of the ethics committee is to provide an opinion before a clinical trial starts, having been given details of the following particulars:

- the relevance of a clinical trial and the trial design
- evaluation of the anticipated benefits and risks
- the protocol
- suitability of the investigator and supporting staff
- the Investigator's Brochure
- the quality of facilities available
- the process for obtaining informed consent and the alternative procedures for doing so on behalf of those incapable of giving informed consent
- details of any indemnity or compensation in the event of injury or death attributable to the clinical trial
- insurance to cover the liability and the investigator and sponsor
- details of payments to be made to investigators and participants in the trial
- arrangements for the recruitment of clinical trial subjects.

Only if the opinion of the ethics committee on all of the above points is favourable will the trial be permitted to start. The legislation requires that the decision from the ethics committee must be supplied within 60 days of the date of receipt of the application. If the ethics committee requires further information to make a final judgement as to its opinion, the time taken for that further information to be supplied by the applicant is not included in the 60-day schedule. For certain products (e.g. medicinal products for gene therapy and somatic cell therapy, or products containing a genetically modified organism), the ethics committee is allowed 90 days to consider its opinion. A further 90 days may be allowed for the opinion of the ethics committee if it considers it necessary to consult further to consider such trials.

To ensure the effective functioning of ethics committees, a new UK Ethics Committee Authority (UKECA) has been created to establish, recognise, establish and monitor ethics committees. The executive procedures of the UKECA are carried out by the Central Office of Research Ethics Committee (COREC).

Ethics committees opinions

The legislation has established a procedure to obtain a single opinion for multicentre trials. If all the sites for the multicentre trial are located within the UK, an ethics committee application is directed to the committee located within or covering an area in which the chief investigator for the trial is based. If the locations of a multicentre trial are in more than one EU Member State, each Member State is required to give an opinion on the acceptability of the clinical trial.

Starting a clinical trial

Before any clinical trial can start, the sponsor must submit a valid request for an authorisation to the regulatory authority of the Member State in which the trial is to be conducted. In the UK, the Competent Authority is the Medicines and Healthcare products Regulatory Agency (MHRA). If the MHRA refuses an application for a clinical trial authorisation, it can be referred to the Committee on Safety of Medicines (CSM) and the Medicines Commission. At the same time as the application to the MHRA, a favourable opinion must be received from an ethics committee (see above). The legislation describes three classes of medicinal product for the purposes of clinical trial authorisations, with varying time schedules for approval of the authorisation:

- general medicinal products
- medicinal products for gene therapy and somatic cell therapy
- medicinal products with special characteristics (e.g. biological products of human or animal origin).

For general medicinal products, the time limit for assessments of clinical trial authorisation application must not exceed 60 days. Extensions are permissible for the two classes of medicinal products other than general medicinal products.

Conduct of a clinical trial

It may be necessary for a sponsor to make amendments to the protocol for the clinical trial. If such amendments are deemed to be 'substantial', the Competent Authority and the ethics committee must be notified in writing. The ethics committee has a maximum of 35 days upon receipt of the proposed amendments to give its opinion. Amendments to the protocol can also be made by the Competent Authority, but before doing so it must give at least 14 days' notice of the proposed amendments to the sponsor.

'Substantial' amendments to a clinical trial or authorisation would include the following:

- the safety and personal integrity of the subjects of the trial
- the scientific values of the trial
- the conduct and the management of the trial
- the quality or safety of an investigational medicinal product used in the trial.

Amendment to the clinical trial authorisation may also be required in the event of the development of significant hazards to the health and safety of subjects that require the sponsor to undertake urgent safety measures. Such actions can be undertaken by the sponsor without prior notification to the Competent Authority, but written notification must follow within 3 days of those actions.

At the end of the clinical trial, the sponsor must notify the Competent Authority and the ethics committee that the trial has ended within 90 days of its completion. If the trial has had to be terminated early, notification to the regulatory authority must take place within 15 days of the end of the trial and the reasons for the early termination clearly explained.

Exchange of information between regulatory authorities

A new EU clinical trial database is to be established whose access is restricted to the regulatory authorities of EU Member States, the EMEA and the European Commission. This database stores the details of the following aspects of clinical trials currently being undertaken within the EU:

- extracts from the requests of authorisation
- any amendments to the request for authorisation
- amendments to the protocol
- a favourable opinion of the ethics committee
- the declaration at the end of the clinical trial
- details of last inspections for compliance with GCP.

Although concerns have been expressed by pharmaceutical companies about the security of such information, the EU database is intended to ensure the confidentiality of all data.

Investigational medicinal products

Manufacture and import

All medicinal products which possess a marketing authorisation must be manufactured according to the standards of GMP and under the supervision of a Qualified Person. Likewise, Directive 2001/20/EC requires that investigational medicinal products (IMPs) must be manufactured according to a separate manufacturer's authorisation. In effect, a pharmaceutical company must possess two manufacturer's authorisations: one for its authorised medicinal products and one for its IMPs. The IMP manufacturer's authorisation covers the manufacture, assembly and/or importation of an IMP. To obtain an authorisation, it is necessary for the manufacturer to comply with the principles and guidelines of GMP as laid down in Directive 91/356/EEC.

If IMPs are imported from third countries outside the EU, the importer must also possess an IMP manufacturer's authorisation. Likewise, where an IMP is manufactured in the UK and is intended to be exported to third countries for use in a clinical trial, the UK manufacturer must be in possession of an IMP manufacturer's authorisation.

Certain exemptions apply to the requirement to hold an IMP manufacturer's authorisation. It is not required if the IMP is repackaged or changes are made to the packaging in a hospital or health centre by a doctor or pharmacist and the IMP is to be used in that hospital or health centre. Equally, the reconstitution of IMPs (e.g. dissolution or dispersal of the product, its dilution or mixing with another substance) prior to administration does not constitute manufacture, and such activities would not be subjected to an IMP manufacturer's authorisation.

The Qualified Person has to ensure that the appropriate test and controls have been carried out on the IMP, and has to sign for each batch to confirm that this has been done. A register of manufacturing must be maintained and entries made into the register as soon as possible after each batch has been manufactured and before it is released for use in the clinical trial. The qualifications of the individual chosen to act as a Qualified Person must be submitted in the application for an IMP manufacturer's authorisation. The Qualified Person must be a member of the Institute of Biology, the Royal Pharmaceutical Society of Great Britain or the Royal Society of Chemistry. The role of the Qualified Person is in effect the same as that required for the control and release of batches of authorised medicinal products.

Labelling

The labelling requirements for IMPs are detailed in Annex 13 of the GMP guidelines, Directive 91/356/EEC. If the product is not correctly labelled in accordance with these requirements, it is a criminal offence for a sponsor to sell or supply or to procure the sale of or supply of an IMP for a clinical trial.

Inspection procedures

The maintenance of the standards of GMP and GCP are critical for the safe and effective use of IMPs. To ensure their maintenance, inspectors are appointed by the regulatory authorities to visit the sites of clinical trials and the manufacturing sites of the IMP. In addition, any laboratory used for the analysis of clinical trial data and the sponsor's premises may also be subject to inspection.

Inspections are carried by a Competent Authority of the Member State in which the clinical trial or manufacture occurs, and the result of that inspection is notified to the other interested parties (i.e. other Competent Authorities and ethics committees) in the clinical trial. This helps to minimise the potential for duplication of inspections by individual Member States. If the manufacturing site or a clinical trial location is in a third country outside the EU, Directive 2001/20/EC provides for inspection by a Member State Competent Authority to be undertaken by appropriately qualified EU inspectors. The inspection report for all inspections is made available to the sponsor and to other Member States, to ethics committees and to the EMEA, should they so request.

Notification of adverse events

Both serious adverse events and suspected unexpected serious adverse reactions (SUSARs) as they occur during a clinical trial must be notified to the

Competent Authority. In addition, the sponsor must also provide an annual list of all serious adverse events (expected and unexpected) and a report of the safety of subjects participating in the trial.

Some adverse events will have been anticipated prior to starting the trial and their details given in the protocol or Investigator's Brochure. However, those not so listed must be notified by the sponsor to the Competent Authority immediately and followed up by detailed written reports. Such reports must be identified by unique code numbers assigned to identify the individual subject. If a death occurs during the course of a clinical trial, the investigator must supply the sponsor and the ethics committee with any additional information they require.

Suspected unexpected serious adverse reactions (SUSARs) that are fatal or life-threatening must be recorded by the sponsor and reported as soon as possible to the Competent Authority and to the ethics committee, and in any case no later than 7 days after the event has been reported to the sponsor. If the SUSARs are not fatal or life-threatening, the report to Competent Authority and the ethics committee must be made within 15 days by the sponsors. The investigators at all sites of the clinical trial with the IMP must also have been notified by the sponsor of the SUSAR.

An EU pharmacovigilance database is to be established for recording all SUSARs notified by the sponsor to the regulatory authority. All Member States will have access to the pharmacovigilance database, but not the sponsors of clinical trials. Other regulatory authorities, the EMEA and the European Commission will also have access to the database.

Fees payable

The regulatory authority charges a fee for the assessment of pharmaceutical, preclinical and medical data for applications for clinical trial authorisations. The fees reflect the time and resources necessary to complete the assessment of the application. An annual service fee is also charged by the regulatory authority to cover proper administrative activities and enquiries related to each programme of trials with an IMP.

Fees are also payable for applications submitted for IMP manufacturer's authorisations, which cover the application, variations and inspections together with an annual service fee during the lifetime of the manufacturer's authorisation. The fee for inspection of a manufacturer is based upon the size of the company inspected as determined by the number of relevant employees. Fees for GCP inspections have also been introduced by the regulatory authority.

References

1. European Commission. *The Rules Governing Medicinal Products in the European Union*, Vol. 3C, *Guidelines: medicinal products for human use: clinical.* Luxembourg: European Commission, 1998.

6

Pharmacovigilance

Pharmacovigilance forms one of the key aspects for maintaining the criteria of quality, safety and efficacy in medicinal products. Once a marketing authorisation is issued, additional information is gathered during the normal conditions of use of a medicinal product. This reflects the fact that the population now using the agent is much larger than that achieved during clinical trials and that the conditions for its use are much less controlled than they were during trials. The requirements for pharmacovigilance apply to all authorised medicinal products, including those authorised before 1 January 1995.

The importance of pharmacovigilance has grown enormously over the last 30 years. This is further made clear by one of the main proposals of the ongoing review of EU pharmaceutical legislation, in which the requirement for the 5-yearly renewal of a marketing authorisation is likely to be replaced by regular updates on the safety and use of a product.

Legal basis and purpose

Like most recent legislation for pharmaceuticals, pharmacovigilance is legally defined by Council Regulation (EEC) No. 2309/93, Commission Regulation (EC) No. 540/95 and Council Directive 75/319/EEC (as amended). The legislation explains the need for the marketing authorisation holder and the regulatory authorities to set up a system for pharmacovigilance for the collection, collation and evaluation of information about suspected adverse reactions. The information received is shared by the marketing authorisation holder and the regulatory authority, with built-in safeguards to prevent duplication of effort, maintain confidentiality, and maximise the quality of the data and systems processing those data.

Terminology

Pharmacovigilance has its own range of definitions and abbreviations, many of which appear, at first glance, to be relatively similar. As a result, precise use of terms is essential to ensure understanding. A list of definitions is given in Table 6.1.

Table 6.1 Pharmacovigilance – definitions

Term	Definition
Adverse drug reaction (ADR)/adverse reaction	An adverse drug reaction in this context is considered as synonymous with 'adverse reaction' and 'suspected adverse reaction'. Adverse drug reaction means a reaction which is harmful and unintended and which occurs at doses normally used in man for the prophylaxis, diagnosis or treatment of disease or modification of physiological function.
	A reaction, in contrast to an event, is characterised by the fact that a causal relationship between the drug and the occurrence is suspected, i.e. judged possible by the reporting or reviewing healthcare professional. If a reaction is spontaneously reported by a healthcare professional, this usually implies a positive judgement from the reporter unless the reporter explicitly gives a negative judgement on the causal relationship.
Adverse event (or adverse experience)	An undesirable experience occurring following administration of a medicinal product. An adverse event does not necessarily have a causal relationship with the treatment.
Company Core Data Sheet (CCDS)	A document prepared by the marketing authorisation holder (MAH) containing, in addition to safety information, material relating to indications, dosing, pharmacology and other information concerning the product.
Company Core Safety Information (CCSI)	All relevant safety information contained in the Company Core Data Sheet (CCDS) prepared by the marketing authorisation holder (MAH) and which the MAH required to be listed in all countries where the company markets the drug, except when the local regulatory authority specifically requires a modification. It is the reference information by which listed and unlisted adverse drug reactions are determined for the purpose of periodic reporting for marketed products, but not by which expected and unexpected adverse drug reactions are determined for expedited reporting.
Data lock-point (cut-off date)	The date designated as the cut-off date for data to be included in a Periodic Safety Update Report (PSUR).
Drug abuse	Drug abuse is persistent or sporadic, intentional, excessive use of medicinal products which is accompanied by harmful physical or psychological effects.
Birth date:	
EU birth date (EBD)	The date of the first marketing authorisation for a medicinal product granted in the EU to the marketing authorisation holder.
	For medicinal products authorised through the centralised procedure, the EU birth date is the date of the marketing authorisation granted by the European Commission (Commission decision date).

continued

Table 6.1 Pharmacovigilance – definitions (*cont.*)

Term	Definition
	For medicinal products granted through the mutual recognition procedure, the EU birth date is the date of the marketing authorisation granted by the Reference Member State.
	For products authorised nationally, the marketing authorisation holder may propose an EU birth date which can be applied to reporting requirements across Member States.
International birth date (IBD)	The date of the first marketing authorisation for a medicinal product granted to the marketing authorisation holder (MAH) in any country in the world.
Healthcare professional	For the purposes of reporting suspected adverse reactions, healthcare professionals are defined as physicians, dentists, pharmacists, nurses and coroners. When reports originate from healthcare professionals other than physicians and dentists, further information about the case should be obtained from a medically qualified person if possible.
Listed adverse drug reaction	An adverse reaction whose nature, severity, specificity and outcome are consistent with the information in the Company Core Safety Information (CCSI).
Post-authorisation safety study (PASS)	A post-authorisation safety study is a pharmacoepidemiological study, or a clinical trial carried out in accordance with the Summary of Product Characteristics (SPC), conducted with the aim of identifying or quantifying a safety hazard related to an authorised medicinal product. Any study where the number of patients to be included will add significantly to the existing safety data for the product, will also be considered a PASS.
Post-authorisation study	A post-authorisation study is any study conducted within the conditions of the approved Summary of Product Characteristics (SPC) or under normal conditions of use. A post-authorisation study may sometimes also fall within the definition of a post-authorisation safety study (PASS). In relation to adverse drug reaction reporting and PSUR requirements, reference to a post-authorisation study means any post-authorisation study of which the marketing authorisation holder is aware.
Reportable adverse reaction – minimum information	A reportable adverse reaction (ADR) requires the following minimum information: • an identifiable healthcare professional reporter (who can be identified by either name or initials, or address or qualification, e.g. physician, dentist, pharmacist nurse) • an identifiable patient (who can be identified by initials or patient number, or date of birth (or age information if date of birth not available) or sex; the information should be as complete as possible • at least one suspected substance/medicinal product • at least one suspected adverse reaction.

continued

Table 6.1 Pharmacovigilance – definitions (*cont.*)

Term	Definition
	The minimum information is the smallest amount of information required for the submission of a report and every effort should be made to obtain and submit further information when it becomes available.
	When information is received directly from the patient (or a relative) suggesting that a serious adverse reaction may have occurred, the marketing authorisation holder should attempt to obtain relevant information from a healthcare professional involved in the patient's care. On receipt of such information the case can be considered reportable. When a patient reports an adverse reaction and submits medical documentation, this should be considered sufficient to be reportable if it provides the minimum information and corroborates the patient's report.
Serious adverse reaction	This includes an adverse reaction which falls into one or more of the following categories: • fatal • life-threatening • results in persistent or significant disability/incapacity • results in or prolongs hospitalisation.
	This also includes congenital anomalies/birth defects and serious adverse clinical consequences associated with use outside the terms of the Summary of Product Characteristics (SPC) (including, for example, prescribed doses higher than those recommended), overdoses or abuse.
	Medical judgement should be exercised in deciding whether a reaction is serious in other situations. Important adverse reactions that are not immediately life-threatening or do not result in death or hospitalisation but may jeopardise the patient should be considered as serious.
Spontaneous report or spontaneous notification	A communication to a company, regulatory authority or other organisation that describes an adverse drug reaction in a patient given one or more medicinal products and which does not derive from a study.
Unexpected adverse reaction	This is an adverse reaction which is not specifically included as a suspected adverse effect in the SPC. This includes any adverse reaction whose nature, severity, or outcome is inconsistent with the information in the SPC. It also includes class-related reactions which are mentioned in the SPC but which are not specifically described as occurring with this product.
	For products authorised nationally, the relevant SPC is that approved by the competent authority in the Member State to whom the reaction is being reported. For centrally authorised products, the relevant SPC is the SPC authorised by the European Commission.

continued

Table 6.1 Pharmacovigilance – definitions (*cont.*)

Term	Definition
Unlisted adverse drug reaction	An adverse reaction which is not specifically included as a suspected adverse effect in the Company Core Safety Information (CCSI). This includes an adverse reaction whose nature, severity, specificity or outcome is not consistent with the information in the CCSI. It also includes class-related reactions which are mentioned in the CCSI but which are not specifically described as occurring with this product.

Responsibilities of marketing authorisation holders

A named Qualified Person for pharmacovigilance must be available at all times to the marketing authorisation holder. If they are not medically qualified themselves, they must have immediate access to a medically qualified person. Details about the Qualified Person must be sent to the regulatory authority in the Member State(s) in which the product is approved and to the European Agency for the Evaluation of Medicinal Products (EMEA) for centrally authorised medicinal products. Some EU Member States require that a local national must also be appointed to fulfil legal obligations for pharmacovigilance. The responsibilities of the Qualified Person include:

- establishing and maintaining a system by which all suspected adverse reactions reported to any of the company's personnel are collected and collated to be available at a single point within the EU
- preparing adverse drug reaction (ADR) reports, Periodic Safety Update Reports (PSURs), company-sponsored post-authorisation study reports and ongoing pharmacovigilance evaluation reports for the national authorities and (where required) for the EMEA
- being able to supply promptly and fully any additional information to the regulatory authorities that is required for the evaluation of the risk/benefit profile of the product.

If the same medicinal product is marketed by two separate companies, each has to fulfil its obligations for reporting safety information to the regulatory authorities.

Regulatory authority responsibilities

As a marketing authorisation issued via the mutual recognition procedure is a national authorisation, the regulatory authority of each Member State must have a pharmacovigilance system in place for that product. For a product authorised by the mutual recognition procedure, the Reference Member State usually takes the lead in pharmacovigilance activities, including the evaluation of reports received by each Concerned Member State and communication with the marketing authorisation holder.

If a product has been approved by the centralised procedure, the European Commission is the legal competent authority. The lead in the evaluation of reports received is taken by the rapporteur originally nominated to assess the marketing authorisation application. The secretariat of the EMEA co-ordinates the supervision of medicinal products authorised within the EU. The Committee for Human Medicinal Products (CHMP) (formerly the Committee for Proprietary Medicinal Products, CPMP) in association with its Pharmacovigilance Working Party evaluates the evidence for centrally authorised products received via the rapporteur. In addition, the Pharmacovigilance Working Party acts as a forum for exchange of information between Member States on all pharmacovigilance issues.

Adverse drug reaction reporting

All suspected adverse drug reactions (ADRs) received from health professionals must be reported. This includes spontaneously reported suspected adverse reactions, suspected adverse reactions from post-authorisation studies, and other reports from the worldwide literature.

If there is a possible causal relationship between the adverse drug reaction and the drug, the term 'suspected adverse reaction' (SAR) is used. Moreover, even if the marketing authorisation holder does not agree with the assessment made by the reporter, the SAR must be reported to the regulatory authority. Only if the health professional does not believe that there is a causal relationship does the marketing authorisation holder not have to make its own report.

All serious SARs reported by the marketing authorisation holder must be followed up and validated. This is the case irrespective of whether the medicinal product was used in line with the information published in the Summary of Product Characteristics (SPC), although overdoses are considered differently (see page 134).

Expedited reporting requirements

Reporting should be made immediately or no later than 125 calendar days from receipt of the minimum information by either any personnel of the marketing authorisation holder or a Qualified Person responsible for pharmacovigilance. If the information is derived from a literature search, the clock starts at the time the report was noted.

For spontaneous ADR reports, expedited reporting is required for both serious unexpected and expected events in all EU Member States. Nonserious reactions are not required to undergo expedited reporting. Serious, unexpected ADRs occurring in other Member States must be reported to Austria, Germany, Portugal and the UK; expected serious reactions are reportable in Germany and the UK.

Content of suspected serious ADR reports and reporting forms

As much information as possible must be sent in cases of serious suspected reactions. The minimum data elements required are:

- an identifable patient
- an identifiable reporter
- a suspected reaction
- a suspect drug.

The internationally recognised terminology (MedDRA, Medical Dictionary for Regulatory Activities) for the details of the adverse drug reaction should be used for the report. The marketing authorisation holder is expected to follow up all such serious ADR reports to try to obtain as much information as possible. Follow-up reports are then to be submitted to the regulatory authority.

Electronic submission of data is recommended using the internationally accepted format laid down by ICH guidelines E2B, MedDRA and standards for transmission.

Impact of reported adverse drug reactions

If the marketing authorisation holder believes that the reported ADR has a serious impact on the previously defined safety profile of the product, this should be indicated on the report form. Such instances may arise if there are a number of serious reports generated at about the same time for the same drug; if it is clear that there is a link between the serious and unexpected reaction and the product; or if the severity, nature or frequency of reactions has suddenly altered. In such an event, it may be necessary to amend the SPC, and the marketing authorisation holder should suggest what amendments it is proposing.

Reporting requirements in special situations

The above information applies to normal use of the medicinal product once a marketing authorisation has been granted. However, serious ADRs may occur at other times, and particular reporting requirements apply in such cases.

Between submission of the MAA and its approval

It is possible that a medicinal product is already authorised in countries other than that in which a further marketing authorisation is being sought. ADRs reported in other countries that might affect the safety profile of the drug should be notified to the regulatory authority carrying out the new marketing authorisation application (MAA) assessment by the applicant company. Whilst it may be difficult to gauge what might constitute a change to the risk/benefit profile, the marketing authorisation holder may be asked to justify at a later stage why it did not refer the matter to the assessing authority.

Use during pregnancy

Reports of pregnancies in which the fetus could have been exposed to a medicinal product must be followed up by the marketing authorisation holder. If an abnormal baby is born the report should be expedited, as described above. All marketing authorisation holders should be on the alert for possible teratogenic effects in the fetus. If such concerns arise, the regulatory authorities of all Member States where an authorisation is held must be immediately informed.

Reporting from other sources

Companies often undertake post-marketing surveys or informal support for patients, and adverse reactions may be notified to them by individual users. However, only suspected serious adverse reactions should be subject to expedited reporting, and dealt with in the same way as described previously.

Compassionate use/named patient supplies

Supply of a medicinal product outside the terms of its authorisation can be undertaken, but ideally under strictly controlled and pre-planned conditions. Those involved in such supply (e.g. the prescriber or the patient) should be encouraged to report adverse reactions to the company and to the national regulatory authority.

Lack of efficacy

A lack of efficacy would not normally be considered a serious problem and should be recorded in the Periodic Safety Update Report. However, with certain classes of medicinal products (e.g. vaccines, contraceptives or those used in life-threatening conditions), its occurrence can be more critical and cases should be subject to expedited reporting.

Overdoses

Expedited reporting to the regulatory authority should also occur if cases of overdosage lead to serious adverse reactions.

Periodic Safety Update Reports

The legislation defines a Periodic Safety Update Report (PSUR) as 'an update of the worldwide safety experience of a medicinal product to competent authorities at defined times post-authorisation.' This review process is intended to assess the information that has been developed since the previous report, integrate that information with any earlier reports, and update the critical evaluation of the risk/safety balance for the product.

The PSUR must be sent to all interested regulatory authorities. For products authorised by the centralised procedure, this would be all EU Member States and the EMEA; for nationally or mutually recognised authorisations, this encompasses all Member States in which an authorisation is valid.

General principles

A single PSUR can be prepared for all authorisations of formulations of a single active ingredient held by a single marketing authorisation holder. If another company has a marketing authorisation for the same active ingredient, it must submit its own PSUR.

If the active ingredient is also part of a fixed-combination product, the marketing authorisation holder(s) can select one of the following: individual PSURs for each of the ingredients and the fixed-dose combination can be submitted; alternatively, subsidiary reports for the fixed-dose combination can be prepared as part of those for each of the active ingredients.

The clinical and nonclinical data provided in the PSUR should relate to the interval since the previous report. The exceptions to this are the requirements to include the regulatory status and serious unlisted ADRs cumulatively since the first authorisation was granted.

The PSUR should concentrate on ADRs: an increase in the frequency of reports is also important information. Proposed explanations for any changes in reporting should also be put forward.

Regulatory status

Cumulative information presented in a table should be provided for all countries in which marketing authorisations have previously existed or still exist. The data should include:

- dates of all marketing authorisations and renewals
- any limitations placed on the authorisations
- indications and any special populations covered by the authorisation
- any decisions and their reasons to refuse authorisation
- withdrawals due to safety or efficacy concerns
- dates of launch and trade names of products.

Frequency of reporting

The period of time between each Periodic Safety Update Report is dependent upon the age of the marketing authorisation. In the first two years post-authorisation, a PSUR must be submitted every 6 months. It is then updated annually thereafter, at the first renewal of the marketing authorisation (at the end of 5 years post-authorisation), and at each renewal date subsequently. An authority can also demand an immediate submission of a PSUR. The PSUR should be submitted within 60 days of the end of the period under review.

The above cycle of submission can be amended with agreement of the regulatory authority. Reasons for this might include new indications for the active ingredient or changes to the dosage form, route of administration or target population.

Reference safety information

Comparison of the performance of a medicinal product over time can only be effectively carried out if there is a sound and agreed basis for that comparison. Most companies produce an internal Company Core Data Sheet, which is usually also the basis for the SPC. The safety information in the Company Core Data Sheet is used as the basis for the Company Core Safety Information, which is used to determine whether, for example, an ADR is already 'listed' or 'unlisted', for reporting purposes. Any changes (e.g. to contraindications, interactions or warnings) made to the Company Core Safety Information over the period of the PSUR should be described, and the revised Company Core Safety Information should be used for subsequent reporting periods.

Data on individual case histories

Information on ADR reports is derived from the following sources:

- direct reports to the marketing authorisation holder
- literature searches
- reports picked up by regulatory authority ADR reporting systems
- others, which include epidemiological databases, reports from poison control centres, and data in special registries (e.g. organ toxicity monitoring centres).

The terminology used to report ADRs in the PSUR should be controlled and ideally based as closely as possible on the ICH terminology to be defined by MedDRA. Many companies have their own ADR dictionaries which are used to describe as rigidly and effectively as possible the range of details reported to them. However, the original description used in a report should be retained on file for future reference, if needed.

Overall safety evaluation

Whilst accurate presentation of the data is important in creating a PSUR, it is only of value if a concise analysis of the data is also given. A review of the experience gained over the lifetime of the product is also necessary, with changes to trends noticed during the latest reporting period particularly highlighted. Significant changes might include new drug interactions, experience with overdose, drug abuse or misuse of the product, and the effects of long-term treatment.

Company-sponsored post-authorisation safety studies

Whilst spontaneous reporting systems can indicate early warnings of potential safety problems with a medicinal product, formal studies can also be beneficial in defining the safety profile of newer products. Company-sponsored studies can be conducted in which the medicinal product is provided by the company, or where the product is prescribed in the usual way in community or in hospital. Post-authorisation studies may:

- identify previously unrecognised safety issues
- investigate possible hazards
- confirm the expected safety profile
- quantify established ADRs
- identify risk factors in the use of the product.

Such studies may be useful in situations where there is uncertainty about the clinical relevance of a toxicological effect in animals, where there is uncertainty about the safety profile, or where there is a highly specific use requiring specialist monitoring. However, these studies cannot be used for the promotion of the use of the medicinal product.

Design and conduct of studies

There are four possible types of study: observational cohort, case–control, case surveillance or clinical trials. In observational cohort studies, the medicinal product is prescribed in exactly the same way as would occur in normal clinical practice. The patient is not specifically recruited into the study but only becomes part of it because the prescriber deems it appropriate for the patient to receive the medicinal product in question. A control group comprises those who present with the same symptoms but for whom the prescriber selects a different form of treatment or different medicinal product. Case–control studies are carried out retrospectively. In these studies, comparisons are made between the product exposure of cases with the disease of interest and appropriate controls without the disease. Case surveillance studies are conducted for those diseases likely to be product-related and to determine product exposure.

The mechanisms of ADRs and the means to prevent them are often investigated using specific clinical trials. Random patient allocation for these trials is normal, and the guidelines on good clinical practice must be followed in these cases.

The responsibility for the conduct of studies resides with the sponsor, usually the medical department of the marketing authorisation holder.

Liaison with regulatory authorities

A draft protocol should be prepared and discussed with the relevant regulatory authorities and independent experts. The protocol, once finalised and agreed, should state the study's objectives, the methods to be used, and the records to be kept, and is submitted to the regulatory authority at least one month prior to starting the study.

Progress reports are required by the regulatory authority, usually every 6 months, which should record:

- the number of patients identified as suitable for the study, the number enrolled, and those followed up
- an estimate of overall exposure (in patient-years, -months or -days)
- the status of all patients who completed the study
- reasons for stopping treatment during the study
- individual listing of causes of death and those hospitalised
- serious adverse events arising.

The usual regulatory requirements for reporting adverse events must be followed and also recorded in the Periodic Safety Update Report for the product. A final report of the study should be sent within 3 months of its completion, prepared according to Good Clinical Practice guidelines.

Ethical issues

As with all trials and studies, the highest standards of professional conduct and confidentiality are required. The patients' right to confidentiality is paramount, and their identity in study documentation must be codified. If patients are approached for information or additional investigations are to be performed, prior ethics committee approval must be obtained.

Pharmacovigilance evaluation post-authorisation

The issuance of a marketing authorisation is recognition that the safety profile of the medicinal product is deemed acceptable at that time and in view of the studies carried out to date. However, the much wider experience gained from the use of the product in a wider and far less controlled environment post-authorisation may require that safety assessment to be revised. If new evidence comes to light which affects the overall risk/benefit assessment, the marketing authorisation holder has an obligation to immediately inform the regulatory authorities.

Risk/benefit assessment

Identification, confirmation and characterisation of product safety hazards in the exposed population can lead to a reasoned assessment of risk. Many different sources of information about the product's use must be reviewed:

- national and international spontaneous ADR reports
- data on ADRs obtained from clinical studies
- laboratory experiments on the medicinal product
- scientific literature
- investigations on pharmaceutical quality
- data on product sales and usage.

An overall assessment of a product's safety can only be made with all the available information.

A reassessment of the risk/benefit balance is required when a new or changing hazard has been identified. The benefit derived from a medicinal product can be measured by the extent to which a disease is cured or alleviated, or the symptoms are relieved; the number of people whose condition improves with use of the medicinal product; and the duration of any response.

Comparison of the perceived benefit with alternative modes of treatment should be made, and a recognition that the level of acceptable risk is dependent on the seriousness of the condition being treated. Greater levels of risk may be considered acceptable in chronic diseases if there is a significant improvement in the quality of life. More serious side-effects and ADRs may be tolerated from a medicinal product used to treat a life-threatening disease.

Improving the risk/benefit balance

It is vital to try to achieve the greatest benefit possible for a patient with a medicinal product when compared to other forms of treatment. Improving the likelihood of benefit and reducing the risks will enhance the balance. Risks can be reduced by increasing the range of contraindications or lowering the dosage. If this or other action is deemed necessary by a marketing authorisation holder, a variation must be submitted. This in turn will necessitate amendments to the SPC and advertising material, whose implementation must be notified to healthcare professionals as important safety information.

Withdrawal of a product on risk/benefit grounds

If, despite any of the changes described above, the risk/benefit balance is deemed to be unacceptable, the marketing authorisation holder has to remove the product from the market. Alternatively, the regulatory authority can revoke or suspend a marketing authorisation.

If the product is approved through the mutual recognition procedure, withdrawal of a product on safety grounds is referred to the Committee for Human Medicinal Products for an Opinion, although the Member State can immediately suspend marketing of the product. For a product authorised through the centralised procedure, the EMEA, the European Commission and all other Member States are informed of the actions by the Member State seeking to suspend the marketing authorisation.

Communication

The notification of the suspension or withdrawal of a marketing authorisation caused by an unfavourable risk/benefit balance must be made to all healthcare professionals within a timescale agreed by the appropriate regulatory authorities and the marketing authorisation holder. For centrally authorised products, agreement with the EMEA is required; for products approved by mutual recognition, the regulatory authority of the Reference Member State must agree the timescale.

7

Medical devices and their control

What is it that links all of the following commonly used items of medical equipment?

- artificial eyes
- dental material and restoratives
- examination gloves
- hospital beds
- resuscitators
- sutures, clips and staples.

Under European Union (EU) legislation that has been transposed into UK law, they are all classed as 'medical devices', and their quality, safety and performance are monitored and controlled in the UK by the Medicines and Healthcare products Regulatory Agency (MHRA). Prior to April 2003, the authority for the control of medical devices was the Medical Devices Agency (MDA). The working of the medical devices section of the MHRA is described in Chapter 10.

Medical devices in effect cover all products, except medicines, used in healthcare for the diagnosis, prevention, monitoring or treatment of illness or handicap. The vast and diverse range of products considered to be medical devices is illustrated in Table 7.1.

The regulatory control of medical devices

The quality and safety of medical devices are paramount, to ensure that their use is effective and safe. Quality and safety cannot be provided by legislation – they have to be built into the design and manufacturing processes for each product – but legislation is required to ensure that standards are applied uniformly and fairly across EU Member States. Most legislation for medical devices is of relatively recent origin, although the UK has had medical device regulations for a considerably longer period.

The first Directive, fully in force in the UK by December 1994, was the active implantable medical devices Directive (AIMD) (Directive 90/358/EEC). It covers all powered medical devices implanted and left in place in the human body. The most common example is a cardiac pacemaker. In the UK, the active implantable medical devices Directive is implemented by the Active Implantable Medical Devices Regulations (SI 1995 No. 1671, as amended) which came into force on 1 January 1995.

Table 7.1 Examples of the range of products legally considered to be medical devices

Anaesthetic machines and monitors	Infusion pumps and controllers
Apnoea monitors	Intrauterine devices
Artificial limbs	Intravascular catheters and cannulas
Artificial eyes	Laboratory equipment covered by IVD directive
Blood transfusion and filtration devices	Lithotripters
Breast implants	Medical textiles, hosiery and surgical supports
Cardiac monitors	Medical lasers
Cardiopulmonary bypass devices	Operating tables
Clinical thermometers	Orthopaedic implants
Condoms	Ostomy and incontinence appliances
Contact lenses and prescribable spectacles	Pacemakers
CT scanners	Physiotherapy equipment
Defibrillators	Prescribable footwear
Dental equipment and dentures	Pressure sore relief devices
Diagnostic X-ray equipment	Radiotherapy machines
Dialysers	Resuscitators
Dressing and wound healing devices	Scalpels
Electrosurgery devices	Special support seating
Endoscopes	Sphygmomanometers
Enteral and parenteral feeding systems	Suction devices
Equipment for disabled people	Surgical instruments and gloves
Examination gloves	Sutures, clips and staples
Fetal monitors	Syringes and needles
Hearing aids and inserts	Ultrasound imagers
Heart valves	Urinary catheters, vaginal specula and drainage bags
Hospital beds	
Hydrocephalus shunts	Ventilators
Incontinence pads	Walking aids
Infant incubators and warmers	Wheelchairs

The medical devices Directive (mdD) (Directive 93/42/EEC) covers most medical devices: from first aid bandages to hip prostheses, and from X-ray equipment to heart valves. Implementation into UK legislation was achieved by the Medical Devices Regulations (SI 1994 No. 3017).

The *in vitro* diagnostic (IVD) medical devices Directive (Directive 98/79/EC) covers any reagent, reagent product, calibrator, control material, kit, instrument and apparatus that is used *in vitro* for the examination of specimens, including blood and tissues from human bodies. Pregnancy test kits and kits for the testing of hepatitis B are examples of IVDs. The Directive came into effect in the UK in June 2000, with a transition period until 7 December 2003.

The CE mark

The CE mark is a mechanism to show that a manufacturer believes that its product satisfies the relevant Essential Requirements in the appropriate Directive and that the product is fit for its intended purpose. It also denotes that the product is considered safe for use in its intended purpose and has been tested to demonstrate this.

Notified Body

Independent assessment of the compliance of a medical device with the relevant Essential Requirements listed in the legislation is carried out by a Notified Body, which is in effect a certification organisation. Once the Notified Body is satisfied that the product complies with the Essential Requirements, the manufacturer can apply the CE mark to its product.

Vigilance and the safety of medical devices

Adverse incidents most commonly arise owing to poor management or inadequate training. Other causes include:

- defects in the design of the device or in its instructions for use
- poor quality control during manufacture
- damage in transit
- inadequate processing, repair or maintenance
- degradation of the device due to overlong use or inappropriate storage
- user error.

The vigilance system

The medical devices Directives (described above) require that manufacturers report any serious or potentially serious adverse incidents to the MHRA. The MHRA shares that information with other EU Member State medical device Competent Authorities and the European Commission if an adverse incident has required corrective action or poses a threat to patient safety. The sharing of the information is intended to prevent the re-occurrence of the incidence or to alleviate the consequences of such incidents. The notification and evaluation of adverse incidents in the use of devices is called the vigilance system.

All manufacturers of medical devices are also legally bound to report to the MHRA any instance when they issue a recall of a device prompted by a risk of serious injury or death through the device's continued use.

An adverse incident may also cause indirect harm to a patient, even though the device does not itself come into contact with the patient. For example, if there is an instrument fault (e.g. in an automated analyser classed as an *in vitro* device), incorrect pathology results (a false negative or a false positive) may be recorded which may adversely affect the patient by their receiving inappropriate treatment or not receiving treatment required.

All adverse incident reports received are acknowledged by the MHRA and the information is entered onto the agency's database. No further action may be required in most of the incidents reported either because the problem was resolved locally or by the manufacturer, or because the report can be linked to an ongoing investigation.

For those reports that are further investigated, the method of investigation depends on the seriousness of the incident. Where there has been a death or serious deterioration in health, an investigation (called a section investigation) is led by one of the MHRA's Device Specialists. The user and/or manufacturer may be visited, the site of the incident investigated, and the device tested – by the manufacturer, the MHRA or an independent test house. Such investigations often result in the release of safety advice by the MHRA.

For less serious incidents, the investigation (termed an Adverse Incident Centre or AIC investigation) is usually carried out by the device manufacturer and its progress is monitored by the MHRA. The person who initially reported the incident is copied all correspondence concerning the investigation and the results of the investigation.

Safety warnings

These are issued by the MHRA to healthcare and social care providers and other users of medical devices. The warnings concern particular problems and risks and recommend appropriate courses of action to minimise these. There are three levels of warning notices issued by the MHRA.

- Hazard Notices are issued following death or serious injury, or where death or serious injury would have occurred but for fortuitous circumstances or the timely intervention of healthcare personnel. They are also issued where it is clear that the medical device caused the incident, and where immediate action is necessary to prevent recurrence.
- Device Alerts are distributed where there is the potential for death or serious injury, or where there may be implications arising from the

long-term use of the medical device. The recipient is expected to take immediate action on the advice issued.
- Safety Notices are used to recommend or inform where action by the recipient will improve safety, to repeat warnings on longstanding problems, or to support or follow up a manufacturer's modifications to a medical device.

Committee on Safety of Devices

A Committee on Safety of Devices has been set up to advise ministers and complement the work of the MHRA. The CSD takes a strategic view of initiatives to make medical devices – and their use – safer and more effective. It also offers advice on the development of device-related policies, advises on the format and targeting of MHRA communications with the NHS, and acts as part of the Quality Assurance System.

The CSD was set up in April 2001 and met for the first time on 19 July 2001. It meets three times a year and the minutes are published on the Internet. A number of ad hoc groups and working parties have been established. The CSD and the MHRA are supported in their work by a panel of almost 100 external experts.

The role of liaison officers

NHS acute trusts, the majority of primary care trusts, and social services department in England have nominated a liaison officer. The liaison officer helps to encourage the reporting of adverse incidents and plays a major role in the dissemination of MHRA safety warnings. The responsibility for the dissemination of MHRA safety warnings to the private sector and to care homes now falls to the National Care Standards Commission.

8

Ethical issues

The primary objectives of all healthcare interventions are to prevent, cure or alleviate disease. Such objectives may or may not be achieved with the use of medicinal products, but the development of medicines for human use does invoke a wide scope of ethical issues that must be borne in mind alongside the basic scientific considerations.

The importance of ethical issues, particularly in the research carried out during the development of new healthcare products, has increased significantly over the last 15–20 years with the greater knowledge and more complex techniques developed, especially in cell biology. The range of tissues now available for experimental techniques for the development of new drugs has increased greatly. Such developments have also thrown into sharp relief the use of animals in medical research, which has always been a highly contentious issue for many people. This chapter focuses upon the toxicological and clinical aspects of the drug development process, and the ethical considerations which must be taken into account at all times.

It must be stressed at the outset that there are no definitive 'rights' or 'wrongs' in the determination of ethical issues: what one person may consider to be an ethically acceptable experimental technique might be viewed as totally inappropriate by another person. Each person will be guided by their own individual morals, and their social, religious and cultural environment. The brief consideration in this chapter of the ethical issues that can arise in the development of medicinal products is provided with the objective of stimulating discussion on these sometimes very sensitive issues.

Historical perspectives

The standards applied to research on human subjects have varied enormously over the course of the past 100 years. It should be remembered that the pharmacological revolution that resulted in the development of vast numbers of new therapeutic agents really only began during the early 1950s. However, research of varying kinds had been conducted for many years prior to that.

Perhaps the worst examples of ethical standards applied to such 'research' occurred during the Second World War. At that time, investigations carried out under the guise of 'medical research' were performed by physicians working for the Nazi administration on members of their own population and on those from countries that had been occupied by the

Germans. Pseudoscientific experiments were carried out on identical twins, on the mentally subnormal and on prisoners of war, each of whom were among the most vulnerable members of society at the time for differing reasons.

Some of those who were involved in these experiments were brought to justice during the Nuremberg medical trials, which brought to light for the first time the horrendous experiments that had been carried out on unwilling and uninformed individuals. Besides the prosecutions that were brought, one major outcome of the trials was the Nuremberg Code, published in 1947, which highlighted the principle and need for informed consent for any participant in a medical experiment.

Much of the impetus for the legislation that controls the development of medicinal products arose from the problems of the use of thalidomide in the early 1960s. The legislation has confirmed the importance of scientifically sound studies into the effects of any medicinal products given to people of all age groups. Society has demanded that the medicines that it uses are of a high quality, are safe and are clinically effective. The ethical basis for clinical research is founded upon the Declaration of Helsinki.

The WMA Declaration of Helsinki

The World Medical Association (WMA) Declaration of Helsinki was originally developed at the 18th WMA Helsinki conference in June 1964. The declaration has gone through a number of revisions, most recently at the WMA meeting in Edinburgh in October 2000. It is based upon and developed from the ethical principles in the Nuremberg Code, but it is not a legally binding document. It does stress, however, that the role of a physician takes precedence over that of the investigator in a clinical trial. The full text of the Declaration is given in Appendix 2.

In its introduction, the Declaration makes the point that 'medical progress is based on research which ultimately must rest in part on experimentation involving human subjects'. It also stresses the primacy of the well-being of the individual subject over the interests of science and society in general. It also recognises that most procedures that are carried out within medical practice, be they prophylaxis, diagnosis or therapy, involve an element of both benefit and risk. It is obviously important to ensure that the degree of risk incurred is proportionate to the level of benefit expected.

In the section of the Declaration covering Basic Principles for All Medical Research, it is stressed that any subjects involved in medical research must be volunteers and must be fully informed about the reasons for the research, its potential outcomes and any personal or other benefits that may accrue to them as participants. The issues concerning the participation of potentially vulnerable members of society are also addressed:

these may include people who are legally incompetent, who are physically or mentally incapable of giving consent, or who may be under the age of legal majority. One further important point raised by the Declaration concerns the use of placebo in medical research. This is especially important because no patient involved in a trial should be adversely affected by their participation, and the potential use of a placebo may prevent that person receiving the appropriate medical treatment for the condition that is being assessed. One of the most important aspects of the Declaration of Helsinki is the fact that it is intended to protect the most vulnerable people in society.

Protecting the vulnerable

Mention has already been made of the unethical use made of those who were most vulnerable in society during the Second World War. Such occurrences have unfortunately been repeated (on a smaller scale) since that time in other conflicts and other parts of the world. One of the groups who are most vulnerable to unethical research are children, for whom appropriate medicines have been produced only infrequently. One reason for this is the tremendous disparity in the responses to a medicinal product between a child of, say, 6 months of age and another aged 12 years. The issue of promoting better medicines for children and the ethical issues that it raises will be discussed later.

Besides children, there are a number of other potentially vulnerable groups of individuals. These groups have been highlighted by a 1995 World Health Organization guideline on the conduct of clinical trials. Vulnerability may be the result of the status of an individual within a hierarchical society or group; through their being placed in a situation where they are not fully aware what is being asked of them as potential participants in clinical research; or due to financial vulnerability as a result of the payments which are often offered in clinical trials.

Those who may be at particular risk from undue pressure from senior members of a hierarchy to participate in a trial include:

- undergraduate students in any healthcare profession, but especially those in medicine, nursing and pharmacy
- personnel working in a hospital or healthcare environment or those working in a laboratory or a nonclinical setting
- employees within the pharmaceutical industry
- serving members of the armed forces.

Those of the last group mentioned above may face a special problem as they are expected to obey orders without question. For enlisted members of the armed forces, failure to do so can result in a charge of insubordination, which is a punishable offence.

Another vulnerable group is formed by those who may have an incurable disease who may be (unethically) persuaded to take part in trials. Such patients might believe that they have been enrolled in a trial for a product which might reverse their terminal illness; equally, they might feel that, as they have an incurable illness, there would be no sense in not participating in something because they have nothing else to lose. Such patients should obviously not be placed in that difficult situation in the first place.

Financial and social vulnerability are also potential problems. Some people may be more susceptible to persuasion to take part in clinical research because of their place of residence or social and financial situation. Examples might include residents of nursing or care homes, and especially those who have little or no contact with relatives or other members of the community outside their local environment. Prisoners, refugees or others who are socially vulnerable may also feel it necessary to agree with 'suggestions' for participation in such research.

The issue of payment for participation in clinical studies has long been a subject of debate. Financial inducements will clearly be of great attraction to those on low incomes or who are unemployed, either with a view to taking part in a trial themselves or enrolling other members of their families (e.g. their own children). When any application is made to an ethics committee to carry out a clinical study using volunteers, the way in which participants are recruited into the trial will be very carefully scrutinised to ensure that there has been no undue or inappropriate pressure exerted on those that have agreed to take part.

Research on prenatal tissue

Many of the most contentious issues in research ethics have arisen within the last 10–15 years following the introduction of new techniques that have allowed research on embryonic and fetal tissue. To understand the origin of such tissue, a brief summary of the fertilisation and gestation period is given.

The origin of fetal tissue

Fertilisation takes place when a sperm penetrates the outer layers of the ovum and stimulates the maturation of the female egg. From the period of fertilisation to 8 weeks' gestation, the fertilised tissue is referred to as an embryo. From 8 weeks to birth, the tissue is referred to as a fetus.

It is important to recognise that fertilisation is a continuous process rather than an event that occurs at a specific time, as fertilisation is only completed between 26 and 30 hours after the initial penetration of the ovum by the sperm. The fertilised ovum is referred to a zygote, whose formation marks the beginning of the development of the embryo. It should also be noted that, although the combination of genes from both the ovum and sperm is complete at fertilisation, the zygote can still split into two or more separate entities up to 2 weeks after fertilisation has occurred, producing twins or higher multiple births.

Cell division begins almost immediately after completion of fertilisation, producing a number of undifferentiated cells called blastomeres. The removal of any of these undifferentiated cells can take place without threatening the development of a complete individual. By the third day after fertilisation, a small sphere of approximately 16 cells has been formed which remains unattached within the uterus for a further 1–2 days. It is therefore at about 6 days after fertilisation that this bundle of cells, probably now numbering 50 or 60, becomes implanted within the wall of the uterus. This process takes a further 12–14 days to complete, at the end of which time a primitive placental circulation has been established. The 'primitive streak', which marks the appearance of the very early nervous system within the embryo, develops at about 15–16 days after fertilisation. It is the generation of this tissue that has formed the basis of the 14-day post-fertilisation limit in legislation in many countries, beyond which research may not be conducted on the embryo.

At the time of implantation into the wall of the uterus, the fertilised ovum is described as a blastocyst. The blastocyst has been formed approximately 5 or 6 days after fertilisation but, in consideration of ethical issues, its importance lies in it being one source of stem cells. The importance of stem cells, particularly in the research into new drugs, is in their potential to develop into almost any other cell type in the human body. They are described as 'pluripotent' as they can develop into many different types of cell, including those of the blood, heart or brain.

Use of the embryo/fetus

Much of the debate about the ethical issues surrounding the use of embryos and fetuses has arisen because of the introduction of *in vitro* fertilisation techniques. In this process, a number of 'spare' embryos are invariably produced. These may be stored and used at some later time for implantation, but a large number of these embryos remain stored and may never be used.

The main arguments about the use of embryos for research purposes focus on the stage in its maturation at which the embryo is perceived to be a non-person or a person. At one end of the spectrum exists the belief that, at the time of fertilisation, another person has been created which has the full rights of a healthy and normally living individual. At the other end of the argument, the embryo is regarded as having no status as a person until such time as there is some brain function. This emphasises the importance of the development of the primitive streak described above.

To further complicate the argument, there is also considerable debate as to the stage at which the central nervous system development becomes meaningful. Should it be at the time the embryo is able to feel pleasure or pain? Should it be at some stage at which the embryo responds to external stimuli? Some people believe that this takes place only very much later during the development of the fetus, sometimes as late as 28 weeks of gestation.

There is also the 'slippery slope' argument, which provides an intermediate view that an embryo or a fetus is not a 'full' person but has the potential for becoming so. In effect there exists a continual process of increased potential for the fetus to become a person, with a corresponding increasing significance and importance attached to that tissue during the period of gestation.

As mentioned above, most tissue is derived from *in vitro* fertilisation (IVF) procedures. At the time of such IVF procedures, far greater numbers of embryos are usually generated than are likely to be used. The remainder are often kept frozen until such time as the donor parents determine that they should no longer be kept or further attempts at implantation are tried. Once there has been a successful pregnancy from IVF, the donor parents are often understandably unconcerned about the fate of the other potential embryos held in storage. What needs to be borne in mind by those who might consider their use unethical is that the further development of this embryonic tissue can only occur if implantation takes place. The availability of these embryos outside the body therefore presents an ideal opportunity for various techniques to be assessed – providing the embryos are less than 14 days old, which the bulk of those that have been stored following IVF generation usually are.

Stem cell research

As previously described, the group of cells formed after fertilisation but prior to implantation is termed the blastocyst. The implantation of the blastocyst into the wall of the uterus marks the beginning of the development of the embryo and fetus. The further successful development of the embryo is very much dependent upon the activity of the stem cells. Their pluripotent properties render them potentially extremely valuable in the treatment of degenerative diseases and this has led to their being cultured *in vitro*. Stem cells can potentially produce nerve cells that might be used for the treatment of Parkinson's disease, pancreatic cells for the treatment of diabetes, and regenerated heart tissue for the treatment of ischaemic heart disease. It has also been suggested that they could be used to generate new bone marrow, lung, kidney, muscle, skin and retinal tissue. Their potential is therefore enormous.

Most currently available stem cells have been derived from human embryos and in particular from those unused in IVF clinics. An alternative method of preparation has been to use cloning techniques that generate a cell line from which the human embryonic stem cells can be cultured. However, their use has generated considerable controversy in many countries. The ethical issues that concern the use of stem cells derive both from their origin in human embryos and equally importantly because of their ability to create and form almost any other type of cell that is found in human tissues.

Research in children

There is a very difficult balance to be struck between almost everyone's concern at seeing an ill child and the fact that, to be able to provide an adequate range of treatments for that child, research must be carried out in children. Traditionally, a medicinal product for an adult has been given to a child at a reduced dose, but often without any clinical research during the product's development into its effects on the younger age group. The reasons why medicines have not routinely been developed for children at the same time as those for adults are varied:

- There is a much wider spectrum of disease and illness in adults than in children with, for example, many adult illnesses (e.g. rheumatoid arthritis, hypertension and renal disease) occurring relatively rarely in those under 16 years of age.
- Children are not a homogeneous group: the effects of a medicinal product on a child of 2 years of age can be significantly different from those produced in a child of 12 years of age. As a consequence, the conduct of clinical trials in those under 16 years presents major difficulties and can sometimes significantly delay the introduction of a new medicinal product to the market.
- Parents or carers are often understandably reluctant to allow their child to participate in clinical trials, significantly reducing the numbers of subjects available to be enrolled in such studies.

Many of the specific ethical issues facing researchers carrying out clinical trials with children have been addressed by Directive 2001/20/EC relating to the implementation of Good Clinical Practice (GCP) in the conduct of clinical trials on medicinal products for human use. This legislation was adopted in May 2001 and aspects of the performance of clinical trials in minors are covered in Article 4 of the Directive.

All individuals taking part in a clinical study, whether they are adults or children, can only take part when they have freely given their agreement to do so. It must be fully explained to any participant why the clinical trial is taking place, what is hoped to be achieved by the trial, and what the role of the participants will be in the trial (e.g. whether blood samples will be required, whether it will be necessary to take tablets or capsules, or whether they will be required to undergo regular medical examinations during the trial). It must also be explained how long the trial will last, the fact that they can withdraw from the trial at any time without penalty, plus any arrangements for remuneration for their participation in the trial.

Clearly, there are difficulties in obtaining this informed consent from children under the age of approximately 8 years. However, it is vital that as much information as possible is still given to children who have some degree of understanding of what they are being asked to participate in, ideally communicated to the child by somebody with expertise in doing so. If the child is unwilling to take part in the trial, that decision must be respected. A request to withdraw from the trial by the child must equally be respected and acted upon.

For children under the age of consent, it is a requirement for the child's parents or legal representative to provide the written informed consent for that child's participation in the trial. The amount of information given to the parent or legal representative should be consistent with that which would be given to any adults who would themselves be participating in the trial.

Society's concern for the welfare of children is also reflected in the Directive's requirement that a trial can only be carried out in children if it is for the benefit of the child and if it is to confirm experimental data previously generated in clinical trials carried out on those who have been able to give their informed consent. Unlike some trials conducted in adults, it is also necessary for the child to be suffering from the clinical condition that is being treated during the trial. Additionally, the trial can only be performed if it can only be carried out in children. All trials should be designed to ensure that minimum pain, discomfort and fear, and other foreseeable risks, are experienced during the conduct. It is vital that the level of risk and any distress caused to the child are monitored constantly throughout the trial.

The European Commission and European regulatory authorities have for some time been concerned about the lack of availability of medicines specifically for the treatment of childhood diseases, and early in 2002 suggested a strategy to try to rectify this situation. It is therefore likely that the number of clinical trials carried out in those under the age of 16 years will increase significantly over the next 5–10 years. Everyone involved in such research needs to be aware of the significant ethical issues and standards under which such trials should be conducted.

Part B

Organisations controlling medicines and medical devices

9

MHRA – Medicinal products

Ask any healthcare professional to name half a dozen healthcare organisations that have a significant impact on the lives of almost everyone in the country: very few (if any) would select the Medicines and Healthcare products Regulatory Agency (MHRA). Even if they could name the agency, it is even less likely that they could accurately describe its pivotal role in UK healthcare.

One reason for this anonymity lies in the fact that the MHRA is a regulatory body – and mention of anything to do with the law conjures up images of dry and dusty texts with esoteric wording and complex interpretations. However, doctors, pharmacists and other healthcare professionals are constantly interacting with and implementing legislation concerning medicinal products and medical devices, making their ignorance of the workings and role of the MHRA less convincing and less justified.

One way to grasp the immense impact that the MHRA has on the general population and on the workings of the healthcare system generally is to consider the issues concerning the supply of medicinal products listed in Table 9.1.

Table 9.1 Responsibilities for medicinal products

Questions
1. Who checks the appearance of and the wording on the packaging of pharmaceutical products dispensed and sold by pharmacists?
2. Who is responsible for checking the wording of the patient information leaflet that accompanies all dispensed and purchased products?
3. The letters PL xxxx/xxxx are printed on all licensed pharmaceutical products. Who issues this number?
4. Who determines whether a pharmaceutical product from a wholesaler can be legally supplied against a doctor's prescription?
5. Does anyone monitor the activities of the pharmaceutical wholesaling companies? If so, who?
6. Does anyone have to approve a clinical trial protocol before a trial can start in the UK? If so, who?
7. Who is responsible for monitoring adverse drug reactions?
8. Who determines whether the safety profile of a marketed medicinal product is sufficiently poor for the indications to be restricted or even to have the the product removed from the market?
9. Pharmaceutical inspectors visit manufacturing sites of pharmaceutical companies. Who authorises the activities of the inspectors?
10. Who checks that the information given to prescribing GPs and hospital doctors corresponds with the approved indications for each prescribed product?

Answer
The answer in all cases is the UK Medicines and Healthcare products Regulatory Agency.

Legislative framework

The MHRA is an Executive Agency of the Department of Health. It was created by the merger in April 2003 between the Medicines Control Agency (MCA) and the organisation responsible for the regulation of medical devices, the Medical Devices Agency. This created a single body for both medicines and medical devices, which mirrors the situation in many other European countries and in the USA. One rationale for the creation of the new single entity was that, in the development of new therapeutic products, there is increasing blurring of the distinction between medical devices and medicinal products.

This chapter will discuss the role of the MHRA in the regulation of medicinal products; its role in controlling medical devices is described in Chapter 10.

The former MCA was itself created in April 1989 (in succession to the Medicines Division of the Department of Health), established on 11 July 1991, and achieved Trading Fund status on 1 April 1993. The MHRA has full financial self-sufficiency: this means that the Agency does not take funds from Government but is supported by the fees it charges industry and others for the services it provides.

Ministerial responsibility for the MHRA is held by the Secretary of State for Health. The Secretary of State determines the policy and financial framework within which the MHRA operates, but does not normally become involved in the day-to-day management of the agency. The Secretary of State is accountable to Parliament for all matters concerning the MHRA.

It is the ministers of the Department of Health who are accountable to Parliament on matters relating to human medicines regulation in the UK. The Department of Health, through the MHRA, discharges functions on behalf of the other territorial health departments in the UK (e.g. the Northern Ireland Department of Health). (Department of Agriculture Ministers carry out a similar function for veterinary medicines, which are controlled by the Veterinary Medicines Directorate, based in Weybridge, Surrey.)

The MHRA is accountable to the ministers in the Department of Health who comprise the 'Licensing Authority'. The Licensing Authority is the legislative entity with responsibilities under the Medicines Act 1968 and relevant European Union (EU) Directives. The MHRA deals with all European legislation that has been transposed into UK law and with which the Licensing Authority must comply.

Functions undertaken by MHRA on behalf of the licensing authority

Medicines are controlled by a system of licensing and conditional exemptions from licensing as laid down in UK and EU legislation. Authorisations to manufacture, market, distribute, sell and supply medicinal products are granted in the UK by the MHRA on behalf of the Licensing Authority (or by the European Commission under the centralised system of approval of marketing authorisations). The MHRA has also been the UK Good Laboratory Practice Monitoring Authority since April 1997.

The MHRA controls clinical trials, advertising and other promotional claims, quality control, manufacture of products that do not have a marketing authorisation, and the supply of imported medicinal products. The safety of medicinal products that have a marketing authorisation is also controlled (pharmacovigilance), and the MHRA is required to take action when adverse effects occur with authorised medicinal products.

The MHRA provides professional assessors and administrative support for the Medicines Commission and the so-called 'Section 4 Advisory Committees' (formed under Section 4 of the 1968 Medicines Act). The Medicines Commission or one of the Advisory Committees must be consulted before a decision is taken by the Licensing Authority to refuse a marketing authorisation or to revoke, vary or suspend a marketing authorisation on grounds of quality, safety or efficacy.

Aims and functions of the MHRA

The aim of the MHRA is to safeguard public health by controlling medicines. The MHRA ensures that the medicines sold or supplied in the UK are of an acceptable standard of quality, safety and efficacy. Equally, the MHRA has to carry out its responsibilities without unnecessarily impeding the activities of the pharmaceutical industry. A detailed list of the functions of the MHRA is given in Table 9.2.

Table 9.2 Functions of the MHRA

- Operates a system of licensing, classification, monitoring and enforcement which ensures that medicines sold or supplied in the UK for human use are of an acceptable standard
- Monitors adverse reactions to medicines and suspected defective medicines, and (where necessary) removes or restricts the availability of such medicines
- Ensures compliance in the UK with statutory obligations relating to the manufacture, distribution, sale, labelling, advertising and promotion of medicines
- Safeguards UK standards for public health protection by representing the UK when regulatory matters are considered by the European Union, by the World Health Organisation (WHO), and in other international fora
- Manages on behalf of the Department of Health the *British Pharmacopoeia* (BP) and work undertaken by BP staff relating to the *European Pharmacopoeia*
- Discharges the functions of the UK Good Laboratory Practice Monitoring Authority (GLPMA)

In practice, the MHRA:
- Assesses new and abridged MAAs
- Issues approvals for carrying out clinical trials in humans for a new chemical entity
- Monitors and varies existing marketing authorisations according to clinical and scientific need
- Assesses and approves changes to the legal status of medicinal products
- Issues parallel import licences
- Monitors pharmaceutical manufacturing sites to ensure they conform to Good Manufacturing Practice standards
- Collects and collates pharmacovigilance reports on new and existing medicinal products and takes appropriate action in the event of safety concerns

The MHRA has declared its intention for new medicines to reach the public at the earliest opportunity. It achieves this by having one of the consistently fastest assessment times in the EU for marketing authorisation applications (MAAs) of new active substances (a mean time of 33 days in 2001).

The organisation

The MHRA is formed of eight divisions whose staffing levels in 2002 are described in Table 9.3. The primary functioning units of the MHRA are the Board of Management and the Operations Management Team. The Board of Management comprises primarily the directors of the agency's divisions and provides support and advice to the chief executive in the day-to-day operations of the agency.

The Operations Management Team (formerly called the Executive Committee) is responsible for the day-to-day operation of the MHRA. Its membership is determined by the chief executive and its purpose is to:

- monitor the performance of the MHRA and deliver the performance requirements of the Annual Business Plan and receive the monthly management accounts
- monitor corporate targets (these include financial targets and business volumes) and receive the Composite Quarterly Report
- develop corporate and business plans for consideration by the board
- review the effectiveness and efficiency of the agency's operations according to a programme of annual priority reviews for each business area
- recommend priorities for the allocation of resources within the agency
- support the culture and communication programme and oversee implementation of human resources policies including the monitoring of training and staff development across the agency

Table 9.3 Staffing levels at the MHRA

Business/area	Full-time equivalents
Directorate	4
Licensing Division	169
Post-Licensing Division	139
Inspection and Enforcement Division	116
Information Management Division	32
Executive Support Division	40
Finance and Human Resources Division	20
GPRD Group[a]	16
Total	543

[a] General Practice Research Database.

- approve and be responsible for the agency's Standard Operating Procedures
- monitor the maintenance of standards and receive reports on quality issues.

The Licensing Division

The Licensing Division is responsible for the assessment of data submitted in support of applications for marketing authorisations.

Licensing Group 1 deals with:

- Assessment Unit 1 for new chemical entities (full and abridged applications) (includes homoeopathics, radiopharmaceuticals, and dental and surgical products)
- Assessment Unit 2 for biologicals (full and abridged applications)
- Assessment Unit 3 for abridged applications
- Assessment Unit 4 for abridged applications
- Committee Support Unit that supports the Committee on Safety of Medicines and its subcommittees
- applications from manufacturers to carry out clinical trials in the UK under the clinical trials Directive
- statistics.

Licensing Group 2 is responsible for:

- the off-site storage of MAAs at Hinchley Wood
- marketing authorisations for parallel imports
- registration of MAAs submitted, data entry and licence issue.

The Biological and Biotechnology Assessment Group deals with the more complex area of registration of biological products and the ever-changing area of biotechnology products.

The logistical management of the receipt of MAAs and the issuance of marketing authorisations is facilitated by a computerised system, PLUS (the Product Licence User System).

The Clinical Trials Unit

The Licensing Division deals with the issuance of authorisations to carry out clinical trials. Formerly the authorisations issued were CTX certificates, issued usually at the beginning of Phase II trials. The Clinical Trial Certificate (CTC) and the CTX scheme were used to authorise the first clinical trials in patients for a particular formulation of a product. Since the implementation of Directive 2001/20/EC, however, all clinical trials must be authorised prior to starting (see Chapter 5), and the Clinical Trials Unit is now responsible for all trials.

Advice to companies

Advice is willingly given by the Licensing Division of the MHRA to companies at any stage during the development of a new medicinal product. In its meetings with companies, the MHRA creates an ad hoc team, whose membership depends upon what the company wants advice about. A full team would comprise a manager, a pharmacist, a toxicologist, a medical assessor and a statistician.

Assessment of the marketing authorisation application

The Division Manager is responsible for ensuring that the work is done within the agreed timescale and for the overall co-ordination of the assessment. The dossier is received in three main parts – pharmaceutical, toxicological and clinical – and each part is dealt with by the respective assessors separately.

To complete the assessment, there are further meetings of the Licensing Division team, particularly concerning the production of individual Assessment Reports for quality, safety and efficacy. From these, an overall Assessment Report is produced, which summarises the MHRA's scientific assessment of the data submitted by the company. It is this that forms the basis for the approval or rejection of the MAA.

The licensing role in Europe

The MHRA is committed to the successful functioning of the European pharmaceutical licensing systems. The Licensing Division has undertaken work on applications submitted through either the centralised procedure or the mutual recognition procedure.

In the centralised procedure, a rapporteur is appointed to co-ordinate the assessment of the MAA. The MHRA is the leading rapporteur (20% of all MAAs) for all centralised MAAs.

Under the mutual recognition procedure for obtaining a marketing authorisation, the principle is that an authorisation is obtained first in one Member State (the Reference Member State). The MHRA is the regulatory authority most commonly used as Reference Member State, primarily because of its highly efficient and rapid assessment.

Parallel imports

The UK Parallel Import Licensing Scheme permits the marketing in the UK of medicinal products that have marketing authorisations in other EU Member States. The sole requirement is that the imported product must be equivalent to the authorised UK product. The administrative procedures necessary for maintenance of parallel import marketing authorisations are identical to those for UK-based marketing authorisations.

Homoeopathic Registration Scheme

This scheme is for use by homoeopathic products that satisfy certain criteria:

- The dilution of the stock contained in the product must be at least 1 in 10 000 of the mother tincture.
- The products must be for oral or external use.
- No therapeutic claims are being made for the product.
- The product name must be the scientific name of the stock.

The MHRA received 44 applications and issued 34 certificates in 1999/2000. In addition, as the scheme has now matured, 34 renewal applications have also been processed.

The Post-Licensing Division

The objective of the Post-Licensing Division is to protect public health by ensuring the quality, safety and efficacy of marketed medicines, including the provision of information to promote safe and effective use.

Post-licensing activities are required for a number of reasons:

- There is limited knowledge about safety when a medicine receives a marketing authorisation.
- As there is a need to make new medicines available speedily, it may be necessary to restrict the initial conditions of the licence.
- The practice of therapeutics evolves over the lifetime of the marketing authorisation.
- Wider access may be safely permitted for some medicines.
- Communications about medicines and their impact on safe use.

The division deals with pharmacovigilance, variations, renewals, legal reclassification of medicinal products, product information and advertising.

Pharmacovigilance

Pharmacovigilance covers suspected adverse drug reaction reports that are submitted via the Yellow Card scheme, Periodic Safety Update Reports, data derived from company-sponsored studies, published literature, signals that may be unrecognised safety hazards, major investigations and, in extreme cases, drug withdrawals. Information may also be received from other regulatory authorities who have recognised a suspected safety issue, and from record linkage databases (e.g. GPRD, see page 168).

Variations to the terms of the marketing authorisation

Variations to the terms of the marketing authorisation may be undertaken for a wide variety of reasons. It is essential that the marketing authorisation holder keeps the authorisation up to date. There may be a change to the indications for which the product is approved, or the manufacturer holding the marketing authorisation may change.

Renewals

A marketing authorisation is valid for 5 years, at which stage its safety status must be reviewed; if it is deemed acceptable, a renewal is issued. The review focuses on the Periodic Safety Update Reports that the marketing authorisation holder has to submit and uses a broad range of sources of evidence on therapeutic evolution.

Changes to legal classification

All new chemical entities are available initially only as prescription-only medicines (POMs). At some later stage in its lifetime, the drug may prove to be sufficiently safe for legal controls on the drug to be relaxed and for it to be made available for sale through community pharmacies. Equally, the safety profile may change in the other direction, with concerns about the safety of a product previously available without a prescription requiring it to be reclassified as a POM. It is the Post-Licensing Division that deals with these legal reclassifications, in consultation with the Committee on Safety of Medicines and following statutory consultation. The final decision is taken by the health minister, following which the POM Order is amended.

Enquiries

A vast number of enquiries are received each year, ranging from those from health professionals and patients to requests for information from Parliament and the press.

Patient information

The division also approves the information leaflets that must be issued with all dispensed medicines. It is assisted in this programme by an MHRA Quality Review Group, which has model leaflets that have been tested on potential users on which to base decisions.

Control of advertising

It is essential that medicines are used rationally and that potential users are not misled by advertising of non-POM medicines. The MHRA in effect monitors the self-regulation of advertising by the industry. All advertising must comply with the marketing authorisation and with the Summary of Product Characteristics agreed at the time of approval of the product. POM medicines cannot be advertised direct to public.

MHRA – Medicinal products

Inspection and Enforcement Division

Pharmaceuticals must be manufactured and distributed to the highest possible standards, and it is a legal requirement that the MHRA verifies that these standards have been met.

The Inspections Group

The Inspections Group covers Good Manufacturing Practice (GMP), Good Distribution Practice (GDP), Good Clinical Practice (GCP) and Good Laboratory Practice (GLP). Almost 650 inspections were carried out in 1999/2000, of which about 60% were in manufacturing sites and 40% at wholesaling sites. All manufacturing facilities are inspected every 2 years, irrespective of size. Inspection of wholesale premises is carried out every 4 years. A small number of GMP inspections are also carried out on behalf of the EMEA. The group also inspects and issues licences to manufacturers and wholesalers of veterinary pharmaceuticals (but excluding veterinary biological products).

The division's Licensing Office is responsible for issuing and maintaining licences for manufacturers, wholesalers and importers. Almost 10 000 export certificates were issued in 2000/2001.

The division takes about 3000 largely randomly chosen samples of both licensed and unlicensed medicinal products for analysis, mainly from community pharmacies.

Examples of unlicensed products that are tested include herbal products. This testing is done to maintain the high quality of medicinal products available in the UK.

The Defective Medicines Reporting Centre (DMRC) receives between 200 and 250 reports each year of potential quality defects, from the public, professional bodies and pharmaceutical companies.

Export Certificates may be issued by the Inspection and Enforcement Division on request to help exporters satisfy the import requirements of third countries. These certificates state that statutory manufacturing requirements have been fulfilled by the manufacturer of the particular medicinal product and that the manufacturing premises have been inspected.

The Good Clinical Practice (GCP) Compliance Unit assesses compliance with GCP guidelines and regulations. To achieve this, on-site inspections are carried out at pharmaceutical sponsor companies, contract research organisations, investigational sites, and other facilities involved in clinical trial research.

The Enforcement Group

The Enforcement Group ensures that there is compliance with medicines regulations. Reports of possible infringements of medicines regulations are received from medicines inspectors, other parts of the MHRA, practising doctors and pharmacists, the Royal Pharmaceutical Society of Great Britain and members of the public.

Marketing authorisation holders may infringe the terms of their authorisations. There may also be instances when people try to sell products for which medicinal claims are made that either have not been or cannot be proven. The group is particularly vigilant in looking for counterfeit medicines.

Laboratories and Licensing Group

The UK Good Laboratory Practice Monitoring Authority (GLPMA) was transferred in April 1997 from within the UK Department of Health to the MHRA. The GLPMA inspects companies that are carrying out nonclinical studies in support of marketing authorisation applications.

Policy, borderline substances, and standards

The Borderline Section determines whether an active ingredient is a medicine, cosmetic or food using an independent statutory review mechanism and a transparent assessment process.

The work of the Policy Group involves giving advice on the interpretation of the legal position in response to enquiries from both within and outside the agency, possibly by producing Agency Guidance Notes.

The Standards Group maintains and audits the division's procedures. Assessment of the division's work is carried out by obtaining feedback from the division's customers.

The British Pharmacopoeia

Production of the *British Pharmacopoeia* (BP) is carried out by the Pharmacopoeial Secretariat Group and the BP Laboratory Unit. The Pharmacopoeial Secretariat Group prepares the BP in collaboration with the BP Laboratory and the BP Commission and its Technical Committees.

Executive Support Group

As its name implies, the Executive Support Group provides the infrastructure and environment in which the agency can effectively and efficiently carry out its activities. It co-ordinates all major policy issues, communications (both internal and external), personnel matters and office support services.

Information Centre services

The Information Centre is the focal point for the information activity within the agency. It deals with information to the public, income generation using information, training in information resources, internal sources of information and published sources.

There is an extensive library and reference collection, and the MHRA subscribes to a vast range of journals. Any press coverage of the activities of the MHRA is also copied and distributed throughout the organisation. On-line databases are regularly scanned, a process which has been revolutionised by the wide availability of CD-ROM technology.

Requests for information come from a wide range of external locations. There is a Central Enquiry Point, which receives about 350 telephone calls each week. Written requests for information are dealt with at the rate of almost 50 per week. Parliamentary questions and ministerial correspondence are also channelled through the Information Centre.

A further activity is the production and publishing of the *Medicines Act Information Letter* (MAIL). The EuroDirect subscription service is also based here, which provides draft and finalised European Union documents.

Fees policy and central support

The Fees Policy and Litigation Co-ordination Unit is responsible for the development and ongoing review of the fees that are charged by the MHRA for the services it provides. Many of the activities essential to the running of the MHRA are contracted out to external suppliers (e.g. reprographics). The Executive Support Division is also responsible for the premises and other office services provided.

European support, policy co-ordination and personnel

The European and Other International Support Unit coordinates all major European and international issues that affect the licensing of medicinal products in the UK. Policy co-ordination by the Executive Support Division may be necessary when a number of MHRA divisions have to provide input into policy advice to ministers, other parts of the Department of Health, and other government departments and agencies. The Personnel Unit deals with all recruitment and promotion issues and induction training for all new members of staff, and gives advice on personnel matters to MHRA managers and staff.

Corporate Services Group

This disparate group comprises personnel matters, facilities and estate management, the building manager, health and safety co-ordination, and the control of the telephone system.

The Personnel Unit operates within a Competence Development Framework, which is intended to improve personal effectiveness, ensure that there are effective interpersonal skills, and ensure that all staff are delivering results and providing a quality service. It deals with personnel and development strategy, ensures that there are equal opportunities for all staff, and manages recruitment and selection and employee relations.

Finance and Human Resources Division

The self-funding status of the MHRA is managed through the Finance and Human Resources Division. The division operates to ensure that all staff understand the requirements of good financial control, the cost of resources, how much income can be obtained from each activity, and the efficiency of working practices in each part of the MHRA. It also aims to ensure that financial aspects are closely allied to all planning of activities, that the financial competencies are strengthened across the agency, and that everyone has the financial information they need to make sensible decisions.

It sets budgets and reports the annual accounts, and deals with ways of controlling income and costs. Almost 60% of the costs are allocated to staff costs, and these and staff numbers are tightly controlled.

General Practice Research Database (GPRD)

GPRD is the most recently formed division within the MHRA. The database was acquired in April 1999 from the Department of Health's Statistics Division and had been previously operated by the Office for National Statistics. It is the largest computerised database of anonymised longitudinal patient records from general medical practice in the world. It currently holds about 35 million patient-years of data.

The data has an immense range of potential uses, including in the following fields:

- clinical epidemiology
- drug safety
- drug utilisation
- health outcomes
- health service planning
- pharmacovigilance
- pharmacoeconomics
- prescribing analysis.

Those who wish to use the database have to pay a fee, a requirement that also applies to the other divisions within the MHRA. Users include academics, the Department of Health, the NHS, the Office for National Statistics, regulatory authorities and the pharmaceutical industry.

The database is operated as a separate function and entity within the MHRA, completely separate from the agency's regulatory functions and responsibilities. It is run on a non-profit-making basis and is also self-financing. This ensures compliance with the terms under which it was donated to the Department of Health. The manager reports directly to the MHRA's chief executive.

The database is not 'complete'. Data is continually being added from about 400 general practices around the country who are paid a fee for the patient records that they supply. GPRD is always keen to increase the number of contributing practices, but already currently receives data from practices that cover about 5% of the UK population.

Information Management Division

The division was established in March 2000 to:

- develop and implement an information strategy
- develop and manage existing information technology systems
- manage information technology systems.

The creation of the Division was in recognition of the vital business and unique importance of information that is held by the MHRA. Its use and release for the full benefit of the Agency itself and for external stakeholders is an essential business requirement.

The existing business process systems are:

PLUS	Product Licence User System
ADROIT	Adverse Drug Reaction On-line Information Tracking
BLIS	Business Licensing Information Services (for inspections)
ECS	Export Certificate System

The Information Management Division is also responsible for subscription-based links for industry to access PLUS and ADROIT. This is done through RAMA (**R**emote **A**ccess to **M**arketing Information) and AEGIS (ADROIT Electronically Generated Information Service).

Information Management Strategy Group

The Information Management Strategy Group is a newly formed group that is investigating ways in which internal efficiency and effectiveness can be improved. Management systems that are being reviewed include finance, personnel, business process and information systems. There has also been a trend to identify new external revenue streams and to investigate finance initiatives.

The other groups that exist within the Information Management Division are the PLUS Management and Development and the ADROIT Management and Development groups.

IT Services

As is inevitable within such a large computer-based organisation, the role of IT Services is crucial. IT Services is responsible for the general maintenance and management of IT throughout the MHRA. It supports and develops various systems that are essential for the successful functioning of the agency's work.

The computer system is regularly upgraded and all the regional offices and Hinchley Wood are also connected to the main system. The major databases used by the MHRA are PLUS, ADROIT and BLIS. There are at least 500 personal computers in Market Towers. IT Services also runs the MHRA's internet website.

10

MHRA – Medical devices

In the UK, the quality, safety and performance of all products classed as medical devices are monitored and controlled by the Medicines and Healthcare products Regulatory Agency (MHRA). The responsibilities formerly lay with the Medical Devices Agency (MDA). The MHRA is tasked to:

'Take all reasonable steps to protect the public health and safeguard the interest of patients and users by ensuring that medical devices and equipment meet appropriate standards of safety, quality and performance and that they comply with relevant Directives of the European Union.'

The MDA itself became an Executive Agency of the UK Department of Health in September 1994. Up-to-date information on all aspects of the work of the MHRA, its structure and functions can be found at www.mhra.gov.uk.

The MDA and the organisation responsible for the regulation of medicinal products, the Medicines Control Agency (MCA), merged as a single executive agency in April 2003. This created a single body for both medicines and medical devices, which mirrored the situation in many other European countries and in the USA. One rationale for the creation of the new single entity was that, in the development of new therapeutic products, there is increasing blurring of the distinction between medical devices and medicinal products.

The main functions of the Medical Devices Section of the MHRA are:

- To investigate adverse incidents associated with medical devices and their use, and help prevent further incidents by communicating findings to those who make and/or use devices.
- To provide advice and guidance on performance and safety aspects of medical devices and their use, to a wide range of customers, stakeholders and beneficiaries of its services. These include device users, their managers and professional bodies; Ministers and Members of Parliament; the Department of Health and the NHS Executive; and manufacturers.
- To negotiate European Union (EU) Directives and implement and enforce UK regulations for medical devices.
- To contribute to the preparation of nonstatutory safety and performance standards for medical devices in support of EU Directives and international harmonisation.

- To manage an external programme to evaluate medical devices and provide consultancy advice, which enable device users and purchasers to select equipment suitable for their needs and contribute to improved equipment design, safety and performance.
- To provide support services for the activities above, including central management; financial and management information; personnel functions and human resource development; and clinical advice.

The MDA was the oldest organisation of its kind in the world, established as a part of the NHS in 1948. As a result, it had accumulated a considerable experience in the standards applicable to medical devices and their evaluation. This gave the MDA a unique international status. However, the MHRA's function has had to evolve to take account of rapid advances in technology, the development of a world market in device technology and manufacture, and the introduction of statutory regulations for the industry.

Until relatively recently, there were no statutory controls on the manufacture of medical devices; such controls as existed were voluntary. As a member of the EU, the UK was one of the first Member States to adopt the statutory unified system for Europe. The UK's long experience of controls ensures that the MHRA is a leading player among EU regulatory bodies for medical devices. Equally importantly, the MHRA has played a key role in developing EU Directives for medical devices, whose primary role is to ensure the safety of the patient.

One of the MHRA's most important tasks is to ensure that those in healthcare responsible for buying medical devices have access to an effective quality control and evaluation service. The Device Evaluation Service provides advice on the quality, safety and performance of medical devices to help purchasers make appropriate choices for their individual needs.

MHRA's primary responsibility is to ensure that medical devices achieve their fullest potential to help healthcare professionals give patients and other users the high standard of care they have a right to expect.

The organisation

The Medical Devices Section of the MHRA is based in offices at the Elephant and Castle in southeast London. Reflecting the diversity of products that are classed as medical devices, there is a wide range of specialities represented among the MHRA's 150 medical device staff, who include:

- chemists
- engineers
- materials scientists
- medical and nursing staff
- microbiologists

- pharmacists
- physicists
- professionally qualified technologists
- toxicologists.

Rapid advances in medical device technology require staff to spend a considerable amount of time keeping up to date. This is facilitated and augmented by the experience and skills of a network of experts in hospitals and universities in the UK and overseas.

Activities are organised into mutually interacting business areas, each with a defined responsibility (Table 10.1). Each of these is considered in more detail below.

Clinical (Medical and Nursing)

This team is the channel for professional communication with doctors and nurses in the NHS, the Royal Colleges and other professional bodies. It is

Table 10.1 MHRA – Medical Devices: business areas and functions

Chief Executive

Clinical
- Medical and nursing advice to all functions of the Agency, the Department of Health, the NHS and professional bodies
- Assessing clinical investigation applications

Device Technology and Safety
- Adverse Incident Centre
- Sterile, surgical and *in vitro* diagnostic devices
- Rehabilitation and transfer equipment
- Wheeled mobility
- Devices for diagnostic imaging, therapy, measurement, electrosurgery and disability
- Critical care devices
- Implants and materials

European and Regulatory Affairs
- Medical devices Directives and Regulations, guidance and enforcement
- Notified Body designation and monitoring
- Registration of medical devices manufacturers and assessment of notifications for clinical trials
- Global Harmonisation Task Force issues
- Global Medical Devices Nomenclature System
- Mutual Recognition Agreements

Device Evaluation Service
- Technical and user evaluations of devices for pathology, diagnostic imaging and life support

Corporate Finance
- Financial and management information

Corporate Services
- Human resources, planning, office services, information systems and library

essential that there is effective and direct two-way communication between the MHRA and practising clinical experts who need support, guidance or information on the safe and effective use of medical devices. The team actively contributes to the investigation of adverse incidents, the evaluation of medical devices, the scrutiny of proposals from manufacturers for clinical investigations with medical devices in the UK, and the negotiation and enforcement of EU legislation.

Doctors, nurses and other users are also given up-to-date information about medical device technology, advising as necessary on the correct use of the complete range of medical devices, including those used in the community.

There are statutory regulations that govern the carrying out of clinical investigations using medical devices. The MHRA has to be notified by the manufacturer 60 days before a device intended for clinical investigation is made available to medical practitioners. Under the notification procedure, if the MHRA does not raise any objections during that time, the clinical investigation can begin. However, objections may be raised if the MHRA believes that there might be a risk to the health or safety of patients and/or users. The MHRA aims to ensure that the notification to manufacturers is achieved as quickly as possible, commensurate with the degree of perceived risk of the device. Clinical investigations with noninvasive, non-implantable devices are therefore likely to be approved more quickly than those to be undertaken with active implantable devices.

A meeting is often held between the MHRA and the manufacturer prior to submission of a notification of a clinical investigation. This helps the MHRA to understand the device and any related problems and for advice to be given about device safety issues and the data to be received in the notification. The manufacturer must show that all aspects of the Essential Requirements (defined in EU legislation) have been addressed in addition to those that are the subject of the investigation.

Notification to the UK Competent Authority (i.e. the MHRA) may be made at the same time as a submission to a multicentre research ethics committee (MREC)/local research ethics committee (LREC). The clinical investigation can begin provided the LREC approval is obtained.

Device Technology and Safety (DTS)

Technically qualified experts in DTS help improve the safety and reliability of medical devices. Adverse incidents are investigated and the reasons for failure are discovered. Guidance for device users is intended to prevent further incidents. It also defines best practice for the use and maintenance of devices so that potential hazards can be avoided.

The Adverse Incident Centre receives incident reports (over 7200 in 2000) and co-ordinates expert investigation into problems. In many cases, a solution is reached with the co-operation of the manufacturer (e.g. by withdrawal of a faulty batch, or by changes to design or instructions for use). In some cases, the MHRA alerts users to a problem by issuing a

Hazard Notice or Device Alert (specific advice for immediate action) or a Safety Notice (information which users need to avoid a potential hazard).

Some incidents occur as a result of devices being used in ways for which they were not designed; others because the device is not used in accordance with the manufacturer's operating instructions; still others because of inadequate training. The failure to understand how to correctly set up infusion pumps has been a recurring problem. Some instances were caused by the use of an infusion pump model with which staff were unfamiliar and had not been given appropriate training. Others were caused by incorrectly setting the infusion rate.

A second group of examples has been the incorrect interpretation of the output from an ultrasound fetal monitor, where the heartbeat of the mother was being recorded rather than that of the fetus, which was subsequently stillborn. These errors have been attributed to likely failure to train users adequately.

In a third example, a patient fell to the floor from a stretcher sling because the buckle straps were not securely fastened. The operators threaded the straps through the buckles from the wrong direction. The straps supported the patient's weight for a short time but, as he was lifted clear of the bed, the buckles suddenly released, dropping him onto the floor. The stretcher had been borrowed from another ward and the operators had not read the instructions or been trained in its use.

Device Bulletins are documents that contain guidance and information of a more general management interest. They are written as a result of experience gained from adverse incident investigations, contacts with manufacturers and users, device evaluations and other sources of information. Recent examples include guidance on blood pressure measurement devices, and information on issues surrounding the re-use of single-use devices.

The experience and knowledge gained from incident investigations determines the advice given by the MHRA to the Department of Health, the NHS and the independent healthcare sector. It also gives the agency an authoritative standing in its dealings with manufacturers and international regulators.

European and Regulatory Affairs Group

The European and Regulatory Affairs Group (ERA) represents the MHRA and hence the UK on all regulatory matters affecting medical devices. This has included negotiating within the EU to create three medical devices Directives which set out safety and performance requirements for medical devices and procedures for checking that products comply with the requirements. Devices that do comply can be labelled with a CE mark. These three Directives have been transposed into UK law as medical device Regulations. ERA works with its European partners to try to ensure consistent interpretation and implementation of these Directives across the EU.

As the Competent Authority for medical devices, the agency has five main functions for which ERA is responsible:

1. Enforcing the Regulations that implement the EU Directives.
2. Providing detailed advice to manufacturers and others on the Regulations. To assist in this, ERA publishes a series of Directive Bulletins that provide a comprehensive guide to the Directives and their implementation and keep the medical devices industry and others in touch with developments.
3. Assessing notifications from manufacturers intending to run clinical trials of their devices, to protect the safety of patients and users.
4. Designating and monitoring Notified Bodies (independent certification bodies which manufacturers use to check that their products comply with the Directives).
5. Maintaining a register of UK manufacturers of low-risk devices and *in vitro* diagnostic devices.

The Device Technology and Safety business (see page 174) is responsible one further function:

6. Operating the vigilance system for adverse incidents reported by manufacturers.

ERA is also active on the international stage: it participates in the Global Harmonisation Task Force which aims to harmonise device Regulations across various trading blocs (e.g. the EU, the USA and Japan). It also is responsible for implementing Mutual Recognition Agreements, in which assessments of quality and safety of a medical device by one Competent Authority are recognised by another Competent Authority. Such agreements have been concluded with the USA, Canada and Australia.

Device Evaluation Service

The MHRA manages a major programme to evaluate medical devices and equipment used for pathology, diagnostic imaging, life support and disability. Most of the work is commissioned from specialists in the NHS and universities.

Devices are tested for performance and safety, as well as technical specification, in both clinical and laboratory settings. The aim is not primarily to identify any potential deficiencies of performance but to provide a clear idea of what the equipment can do, its ease of use and its suitability for different environments and applications.

Over three million people in Britain depend on disability equipment, including wheelchairs, artificial limbs, walking aids and equipment for daily living. The agency's Blackpool Unit has specialised equipment for testing wheelchairs and artificial limbs to European or international standards. It also uses its laboratory to support adverse incident investigations and the development of standards.

The evaluation programme provides a range of service, including consultancy advice, published reports and comparative surveys. These services enable device users to select equipment suitable for their needs, provide information to purchasers of supplies and contribute to improved equipment design and performance. About 100 evaluation reports are published each year. The range of recent reports illustrates the diversity of the evaluation programme's work: they have included anaesthetic workstations, defibrillators, infusion pumps, magnetic resonance and computed tomography scanners, wheelchairs and moving and handling equipment.

The reports provide users with an objective appraisal when selecting equipment for purchase. They also offer essential information to anyone involved in the design, production and testing of medical devices.

11

The EMEA – Supranational drug regulation

Chapters 9 and 10 explain the role of the Medicines and Healthcare products Regulatory Agency (MHRA) in the control of medicinal products and medical devices, respectively, in the UK. A further way in which medicinal products can be approved for use in the UK is through the centralised procedure, with assessment of a product's quality, safety and efficacy by the European Agency for the Evaluation of Medicinal Products (EMEA).

Thirty years after the introduction of the first European Community Directive on the control of pharmaceuticals across the Community (Directive 65/65/EEC),[1] a pan-European regulatory authority was established on 1 February 1995. The EMEA became the first regulatory authority in Europe, and indeed globally, that was empowered to assess marketing authorisation applications (MAAs) for human and veterinary medicinal products beyond national boundaries. The legislative framework created by the bodies and institutions of the EU permitted the issuance of a single marketing authorisation by the European Commission valid across all Member States. The EMEA assesses MAAs for medicinal products, and the marketing authorisation is then issued by the European Commission. Once approved, the products can be sold and used by all 480 million people in the EU.

The legal framework of the EMEA

Council Regulation (EEC) No. 2309/93 of 23 July 1993[2] led to the creation of the EMEA. An EU Regulation can be proposed by the European Council or the European Commission. When it is passed, it becomes immediately effective in all Member States without national legislation having to be created in each Member State. Council Regulation (EEC) No. 2309/93 created the centralised procedure for the approval of MAAs of innovative medicinal products (for which its use is optional) and of products derived from biotechnology (for which its use is mandatory). The assessment and approval procedure of medicinal products submitted through the centralised procedure is co-ordinated by the EMEA. Scientific assessment of human medicinal products is carried out by the Committee for Proprietary Medicinal Products (assessment of veterinary medicinal products is carried out by the Committee for Veterinary Medicinal Products).

EC heads of state and governments chose London as the seat of the EMEA on 29 October 1993, despite many other European cities expressing a desire to be the agency's home. The EMEA is located in the east end of London, in Canary Wharf, between the City of London and the London City Airport. Its contact details are:

> EMEA
> 7 Westferry Circus
> Canary Wharf
> London E14 4HB
> United Kingdom
> Tel: +44 (0)20 7418 8400
> Fax: +44 (0)20 7418 8416
> e-mail: mail@emea.eudra.int
> web site: www.emea.eu.int

Review of pharmaceutical legislation

In considering the current structure and roles of the EMEA and its scientific committees, it is important to be aware that a review of pharmaceutical legislation, and hence of the Agency and its committees, has been under way since 2000. This review was scheduled by the original Regulation to take place within 6 years of that Regulation coming into force. That the review would be required was recognition of the rapidly developing scientific environment in which medicinal products are being developed (particularly in the fields of biotechnology) and the changing marketplace (especially the trend towards globalisation of the pharmaceutical industry).

An audit of the EMEA's procedures and operations was started early in 2000 and was completed in January 2001. The review of pharmaceutical legislation being carried out by the European Commission takes account of the outcomes of the audit and has the following objectives:

- To guarantee a high level of health protection for European citizens, in particular making safe, innovative products available to patients as quickly as possible.
- To guarantee tighter surveillance of the market, in particular by strengthening pharmacovigilance procedures.
- For veterinary medicinal products, to improve the level of animal health, in particular by increasing the number of medicinal products available.
- To complete the internal market for pharmaceuticals while taking globalisation into account.
- To set up a legal framework that fosters the competitiveness of the European industry.
- To meet the challenges of enlargement of the European Union.

- To take the opportunity to rationalise and if possible simplify the system (thereby achieving better regulation), to improve its overall consistency, its profile and the transparency of decision-making procedures.

A new Regulation has been drafted, and the main changes that it proposes are explained below in the description of the current structure and functions of the EMEA and its committees.

The structure of the EMEA

The EMEA currently comprises an Executive Director, a Management Board, three scientific committees and a secretariat. The three committees are the Committee for Proprietary Medicinal Products (CPMP), the Committee for Veterinary Medicinal Products (CVMP) and the Committee for Orphan Medicinal Products (COMP).

Management Board

Currently the Management Board consists of two representatives from each Member State; two representatives of the European Commission; and two representatives appointed by the European Parliament. The chairman and vice-chairman of the board are elected from among its members for a 3-year term of office. The Management Board usually meets four times a year and is responsible, amongst other activities, for agreeing the EMEA's Work Programme for each year and adopting the budget for the agency.

Under the proposed revision of EU pharmaceutical legislation, the Management Board will consist of 16 members, divided equally between the following four groups: representatives of Member States, of the European Parliament, of the European Commission, and of patients and industry, all appointed by the Commission.

An Advisory Board is also to be created, which will consist of one representative of each of the national authorities competent in the authorisation of human and veterinary medicinal products. Meetings of the Advisory Board can also be attended by the Executive Director and by members of the European Commission. The Advisory Board can be sent questions about any aspect of the procedures for authorisation of medicinal products by the Commission, although its opinions are not binding in any way.

Scientific committees

The scientific committees are responsible for preparing the agency's Opinions on any issue relating to human medicinal products (CPMP) and veterinary medicinal products (CVMP). The COMP has also recently been formed.

Executive Director

An Executive Director is appointed, usually for a period of 5 years, although this may be extendable. The first Executive Director came from France; the current (2004) Executive Director is from Sweden.

Secretariat

The Secretariat has recently been reorganised into the following units:

- Directorate
- Financial Controller
- Pre-authorisation Evaluation of Medicines for Human Use
- Post-authorisation Evaluation of Medicines for Human Use
- Veterinary Medicines and Inspections
- Communications and Networking
- Administration.

Activities of the EMEA

The EMEA has published a Mission Statement and a summary of its Main Tasks (Table 11.1).

Table 11.1 Mission statement and main tasks of the EMEA

The European Agency for the Evaluation of Medicinal Products
Directory, 1 January 1999, London, 1999

EMEA mission statement
To contribute to the protection and promotion of public and animal health by:
- Mobilising scientific resources from throughout the European Union to provide high quality evaluation of medicinal products, to advise on research and development programmes and to provide useful and clear information to users and health professionals.
- Developing efficient and transparent procedures to allow timely access by users to innovative medicines through a single European marketing authorisation.
- Controlling the safety of medicines for humans and animals, in particular through a pharmacovigilance network and the establishment of safe limits for residues in food-producing animals.

Main tasks of the EMEA
- Provide the Member States and the Community institutions with the best possible scientific advice on questions concerning quality, safety and efficacy of medicinal products for human and veterinary use.
- Establish a multinational scientific expertise through the mobilisation of existing national resources in order to achieve a single evaluation via a centralised or decentralised marketing authorisation system.
- Organise speedy, transparent and efficient procedures for the authorisation, surveillance and, where appropriate, withdrawal of products in the European Union.
- Advise companies on the conduct of pharmaceutical research.
- Reinforce the supervision of existing medicinal products in coordinating national pharmacovigilance and inspection activities.
- Create the necessary databases and telecommunication facilities to promote a more rational drug use.

Evaluation of medicinal products for human use

Administrative structure

Upon creation of the EMEA a single unit, the Unit for Evaluation of Medicinal Products for Human Use, was formed to deal with all matters affecting medicinal products for human use. In January 2001, however, this unit was split in two, to create the Unit for the Pre-authorisation Evaluation of Medicines for Human Use and the Unit for the Post-authorisation Evaluation of Medicines for Human Use.

The Unit for the Pre-authorisation Evaluation of Medicines for Human Use has three sectors, dealing with scientific advice and orphan drugs; quality of medicines; and safety and efficacy of medicines. The Unit for the Post-authorisation Evaluation of Medicines for Human Use comprises two sectors: regulatory affairs and organisational support; and pharmacovigilance and post-authorisation safety and efficacy of medicines.

The main scientific work for medicinal products for human use is carried out by the CPMP. Under the review of pharmaceutical legislation (see page 180), this committee is to be renamed more logically as the Committee for Human Medicinal Products (CHMP), and its membership is to be modified from two representatives from each Member State to one per Member State. The opportunity to co-opt members will also be introduced to ensure that the necessary scientific representation is maintained.

Assessment of marketing authorisation applications

The primary activity of the Unit for the Pre-authorisation Evaluation of Medicines for Human Use, through its two scientific committees, is the assessment of MAAs for new medicinal products and new active substances. In carrying out the assessment, the scientific committee concerned (either the CPMP or the COMP) produces an Opinion which is then transmitted to the European Commission for conversion into a legally binding Decision (i.e. approval).

In 2001, the EMEA received 110 applications, of which 58 were for new medicinal products and 40 for new active substances. The remaining 12 applications were for products to be approved under orphan drug legislation. Under EU legislation, an MAA submitted via the centralised procedure to the EMEA should take a maximum of 210 days to be assessed. All the applications were assessed in 2001 within an average of 170 days, a timescale that does not include the time taken for the agency to ask questions and receive responses from applicant companies.

A further average of 76 days has been required for the conversion of the Opinion into a Decision by the European Commission, and is the one aspect of the centralised procedure that has received greatest criticism. Attempts are being made to minimise the delays in the decision-making process.

Variations

Once a marketing authorisation is approved, there can arise the need to change various aspects of the terms of the authorisation. This is achieved by a variations procedure, with relatively simple changes to the authorisation (e.g. changes to the manufacturing process) classed as Type I variations. More fundamental changes to the terms of the authorisation are termed Type II variations and are often related to safety issues arising from the use of a new medicinal product. In 2001, the EMEA received nearly 450 Type I variations and more than 250 Type II variations.

Pharmacovigilance

All marketing authorisation holders are required to report adverse drug reactions (ADRs) to their products to the EMEA. All ADRs, whether they occur inside or outside the EU, must be reported. In 2001, there were 20 000 reports from outside the EU and more than 14 000 from within the EU.

Scientific advice

Companies are encouraged to seek scientific advice from the EMEA's scientific committees at any stage during the development process prior to submission of the MAA. Under the legislation, a formal advice letter should be given to the enquirer within 120 days of the initial request for assistance. The CPMP has a Scientific Advice Review Group for this purpose, which in 2001 gave formal advice on 65 occasions. More than two-thirds of all requests for advice relate to the clinical aspects of the development process, and in particular to the performance of Phase III clinical trials.

Under the review of pharmaceutical legislation, a standing working party is to be created attached to the CHMP. This will be responsible for the development and adoption of scientific opinions and the provision of advice to companies. This proposal is considered to be of particular value to small and medium-sized companies that are developing biotechnology products or completely new therapies.

Arbitration and community referrals

The EMEA is primarily concerned with the assessment of medicinal products by the CPMP through the centralised procedure. However, CPMP is also legislatively required to become involved in disputes involving the mutual recognition procedure (by which a marketing authorisation valid in one Member State should be approved by any other Member State in which the marketing authorisation holder wishes to market its product). The legislative basis for such disputes is either Article 10 of Directive 75/319/EEC or Article 11 of the same Directive.

Under Article 10, CPMP is asked to arbitrate on a disagreement between Member States on a medicinal product within the mutual recognition procedure. In 2001, there were six such examples either completed or on-going. Article 11 referrals are made when the conditions of a marketing authorisation (usually the indications approved) are being harmonised throughout the EU. There were nine such referrals made during 2001.

Further information on this activity is given below under the work of the Mutual Recognition Facilitation Group of the CPMP.

International activities

Another important aspect of the work of the EMEA and its scientific committees is the ongoing process to harmonise the requirements for the registration of pharmaceuticals in all the major global markets (the EU, the USA and Japan). The ICH process (the International Conference for the Harmonisation of the Technical Requirements for the Registration of Pharmaceuticals for Human Use) has been ongoing for some years (see Chapter 13) and the EMEA and its scientific committees have played an important role in its activities. The work promoted by the ICH process not only enables tripartite developments to take place but also enhances the work of bilateral negotiations (e.g. those carried out between the EMEA and the US Food and Drug Administration under the auspices of the US-EU Trans-Atlantic Business Dialogue).

Other drug control organisations with which the EMEA has conducted bilateral discussions include the World Health Organization (WHO) Collaborating Centre for International Drug Monitoring, the WHO International Non-proprietary Name (INN) programme, and the Canadian authority, Health Canada.

Orphan medicinal products

'Orphan medicinal products' are used for the diagnosis, prevention or treatment of life-threatening or serious conditions that occur only rarely and affect not more than 5 in 10 000 people in the EU. Under normal circumstances, the high costs associated with the development of new medicinal products would preclude the likelihood of pharmaceutical companies generating a profit from developing medicinal products for such conditions. The EU has therefore followed the example set by the USA in passing orphan drug legislation, through which incentives are offered to companies that carry out research and development to produce medicinal products for such rare conditions.

The incentives that have been agreed under Regulation (EC) No. 141/2000 are:

- Market exclusivity will be given for 10 years after the granting of a marketing authorisation (i.e. during that period, directly competitive similar products cannot usually be placed on the market).

- The provision of scientific advice from the EMEA to facilitate the development of the medicinal product, and guidance on preparing an MAA that will satisfy regulatory requirements. This will maximise the company's chances of getting the medicinal product approved.
- Direct access to the centralised procedure, allowing the approved product to be marketed in all EU Member States.
- Reduced fees are offered for both scientific advice and the submission of the MAA, using subsidised funds from the European Commission that have been agreed annually by the European Parliament.
- There may be financial assistance to companies and organisations developing orphan medicinal products through grants from Community and Member State programmes and initiatives supporting research and development, including the Community framework programmes.

Designation of a product as an orphan drug and its assessment is carried out within the EMEA by the Committee for Orphan Medicinal Products (COMP). COMP has one representative nominated by each Member State, plus three from patient organisations and three from the EMEA.

COMP has 90 days in which to approve (or otherwise) a request for orphan drug designation; a positive Opinion on the designation is then forwarded to the European Commission, which has a further 30 days in which to confirm the Opinion and issue a Decision. Once this is completed, the medicinal product is placed on the Register of Orphan Medicinal Products.

In the early period of the operation of COMP, most of the medicinal products that were granted orphan drug status were for the treatment of cancers, immunological diseases, and metabolic diseases often related to enzyme deficiencies. Equally importantly, about two-thirds of the products were for the treatment of children, drugs for whom have traditionally been a group to which pharmaceutical companies have been reluctant to devote time and resources owing to the relatively small potential market. Examples of medicinal products that have been designated as orphan medicinal products since 2000 are given in Table 11.2.

Working parties and ad hoc groups

Much of the work of the EMEA and the CPMP is carried out away from the main committee, utilising experts from around the EU to provide advice and develop guidelines for the industry on specific topics. A number of working parties and ad hoc groups have been formed. These meet either each month, or at various intervals throughout the year. Each produces an annual report of its activities, which is usually presented to the CPMP. Examples of current and former working parties and ad hoc groups include:

- Biotechnology Working Party
- Efficacy Working Party
- Safety Working Party

- Pharmacovigilance Working Party
- Joint CVMP/CPMP Quality Working Party
- Ad hoc Working Group on Blood Products
- Herbal Medicinal Products Working Party.

Each of these working parties produces guidance documents and ensures that previously generated documents are kept up to date. The activities of the Herbal Medicinal Products Working Party is likely to be superseded in the near future by a fourth main scientific committee, the Committee on Herbal Medicinal Products, which has been proposed under the revision of pharmaceutical legislation.

CPMP satellite groups

Other activities that have been undertaken alongside those of the main work of the CPMP include an Invented Names Review Group, the CPMP

Table 11.2 Examples of medicinal products that have been designated orphan medicinal products under Regulation (EC) No. 141/2000 since 2000

Medicinal product	Condition to be treated
Azacitidine	Myelodysplastic syndromes
Bryostatin-1	Oesophageal cancer
Carmustine (solution for intratumoural injection)	Glioma
Colistimethate sodium	*Pseudonomas aeruginosa* lung infection (including colonisation) in cystic fibrosis
Eflornithine hydrochloride	Familial adenomatous polyposis (FAP)
Epothilone b	Ovarian cancer
Fumagillin	Diarrhoea associated with intestinal microsporidial infection
Granulocyte–macrophage colony-stimulating factor receptor antagonist	Juvenile myelomonocytic leukaemia
Human transferrin conjugated to mutant diphtheria toxin	Glioma
Miltefosine	Visceral leishmaniasis
Mitotane	Adrenal cortical carcinoma
Myristoylated-peptidyl-recombinant scr1-3 of human complement receptor type i	Prevention of post-transplantation graft dysfunction
Pseudomonas exotoxin (domains ii/iii) – interleukin-13 chimeric protein	Glioma
Purified bromelain	Partial deep dermal and full-thickness burns
Thymalfasin	Hepatocellular carcinoma

Organisational Matters Group (ORGAM), and the meetings of the chairmen of CPMP and working parties. The Invented Names Review Group was established in November 1999. It tries to maintain consistency in the review of invented names proposed by applicants from a safety and public health perspective, and operates to update the guideline currently operational for the choice of proprietary names for products that are authorised through the centralised procedure. The group comprises representative of Member States, the European Commission and the EMEA.

ORGAM was created to develop guidance for use both within and outside the EMEA on procedural issues in the operations of the CPMP and the centralised procedure. Amongst other issues, it has investigated the accelerated review procedure and the conduct of oral explanations by applicant companies.

One of the problems of operating and working within an entity as disparate as the EMEA is knowing what is going on in all the other parts of the organisation. To try to ensure that there is sufficient multi-disciplinary interaction in all its activities, the chairman and vice-chairman of the CPMP and the chairmen of CPMP's working parties meet, with EMEA representatives, to discuss current and future activities.

CPMP and COMP ad hoc working groups

Ad hoc working groups may be formed to deal with issues as they arise, either in the working of the CPMP or from external sources. Under CPMP, some of the topics for which ad hoc groups have been convened include oncology, comparability of biotechnology products, paediatrics and pharmacogenetics. Ad hoc groups that have been formed by COMP include the Biotechnology Working Party and the Working Group on Epidemiology.

Mutual recognition facilitation group

As part of its remit, CPMP arbitrates on issues that arise during the mutual recognition approval system. A relatively small number (less than 1%) of MAAs and variation applications submitted in one Member State provoke referrals by a second Member State to the CPMP. For details of the types of activities undertaken by the Mutual Recognition Facilitation Group, see Arbitration and Community Referrals on page 184.

Guidance documents on the use of the mutual recognition procedure have been prepared by the group. Topics covered include national administrative processes in the mutual recognition procedure and a best-practice guide for renewals under the mutual recognition procedure. A Joint CPMP/Mutual Recognition Facilitation Group Working Party has been created to promote the preparation of harmonised Summaries of Product Characteristics (SPCs) for a range of medicinal products.

Evaluation of veterinary medicinal products

The EMEA Unit for Veterinary Medicines and Inspections deals with the assessment of MAAs under the centralised procedure through the work of the Committee for Veterinary Medicinal Products (CVMP). A number of working parties and ad hoc groups also assist in this work.

Assessment of marketing authorisation applications

There are a relatively small number of veterinary MAAs each year: 10 were submitted in 2001, of which nine were for new and innovative products. Applications for maximum residue limits (MRLs) for veterinary medicinal products for food animals are also made to CVMP, though again in relatively small numbers (five in 2001).

CVMP activities

CVMP usually meets 11 times a year (there are no meetings normally scheduled for August); it has also established a Strategic Planning Group to assist in a range of issues, including the fairer allocation of rapporteurs and co-rapporteurs, the training of assessors and compliance with post-authorisation obligations. Pre-submission meetings with companies are held for almost all veterinary MAAs.

Establishment of MRLs for older products

Although all new products must have a current MRL, older products approved prior to the introduction of the MRL regulation still await definitive determination. The work of the CVMP in establishing definitive MRLs for older products means that there are now relatively few products that remain to be assessed.

Post-authorisation activities

In common with medicinal products for human use, manufacturers of veterinary medicinal products can seek to extend the range of indications that are approved, or to amend the marketing authorisation by the submission of variations. Such line extensions and variations are assessed by CVMP, and the number of such applications continues to increase with the increasing number of centrally approved veterinary medicinal products.

MRLs can also be updated and their approval extended to cover additional species. One of the more common changes requested is to allow minor species also to be covered under MRLs that are normally initially approved for major species.

Pharmacovigilance and maintenance activities

Monitoring of ADRs reported for veterinary medicinal products is carried out by the CVMP Pharmacovigilance Working Party. Each marketing authorisation holder has to submit periodic safety update reports (PSURs) for centrally authorised products.

Other activities

CVMP, like CPMP, is tasked with resolving arbitration and Community referrals (see above) for veterinary medicinal products submitted through the mutual recognition procedure. The legislative bases for referrals for veterinary products are Articles 18 and 20 of Council Directive 85/851/EEC. A Veterinary Mutual Recognition Facilitation Group also assists CVMP in this work.

CVMP can also offer scientific advice to companies prior to submission of MAAs.

Working parties and ad hoc groups

Working parties and ad hoc groups have been created to deal with specific topics and issues. In particular the working parties draft guidelines and assist in workshops between the regulatory authority, veterinary trade organisations and companies.

Under CVMP, the following working parties and ad hoc groups exist:

- Efficacy Working Party
- Immunologicals Working Party
- Pharmacovigilance Working Party
- Safety Working Party
- Joint CPMP/CVMP Working Party
- Ad hoc group on Microbial Resistance.

Inspections

When originally created, the Sector for Inspections was part of the Technical Co-ordination Unit. Under the reorganisation of the EMEA's structure in 2001, it became part of the Unit for Veterinary Medicines and Inspections.

Co-ordination of inspections for centralised procedure

Inspections to ensure compliance with Good Manufacturing Practice (GMP) are carried out both before and after the issue of a centralised marketing authorisation. Much of the information on inspections is stored on a centralised database. There is a joint audit programme to harmonise the conduct of inspections, the quality of defect reports, and authorisation of manufacturing sites through quality audits of inspection services.

Good Clinical Practice (GCP) inspections are also carried out for human medicinal products, which involve sponsor companies, investigators and laboratory sites within and outside the EU. Compliance with post-authorisation activities (e.g. pharmacovigilance) may be carried out at some sites at the same time.

Mutual recognition agreements

To make the most efficient use of available resources, a number of countries have implemented mutual recognition agreements by which inspectors from one country can perform inspections locally on behalf of another country. Such agreements have been implemented or proposed between the EU and Australia, New Zealand, Canada, the USA, Switzerland and Japan. Some cover human medicinal products only; others cover both human and veterinary medicinal products.

Certification of medicinal products

More than 12 000 certificates were issued for medicinal products during 2001, which places a large administrative burden on the system. An information package is available to provide guidance on the certification of medicinal products in the EU.

Administration and support activities

All internal services that support the other activities of the EMEA are organised by the Administration Unit. Sectors cover personnel and budget, infrastructure services and accounting.

Administration

The personnel budget for the approximately 250 EMEA staff for 2002 was €28.6 million, which accounts for approximately 40% of the total agency revenue. Allocations of staff for 2002 to each unit are shown in Table 11.3. Staff originate from all EU Member States except Luxembourg, with the greatest proportion (more than 20%) coming from the UK. France and Germany account for about one-quarter of the remaining staff.

Running a large organisation with such a large proportion of its work carried out by external experts and committee members requires efficient facilities management, archiving, reprographics and mailroom services. Office meeting space is also very important, and extensive conference facilities are available on the third floor of the Canary Wharf building.

Table 11.3 EMEA staff allocations per unit in 2002

Unit	Staff
Directorate and financial control	11
Pre-authorisation Evaluation of Medicines for Human Use	57
Post-authorisation Evaluation of Medicines for Human Use	61
Veterinary Medicines and Inspections	36
Communication and Networking	46
Administration	39
Additional posts in general reserve	1
Total	251

Budgetary constraints have been imposed on the agency, with a more or less fixed proportion of its income coming from the European Commission, despite increasing activities and responsibilities. Upon its creation in 1995, approximately 80% of the EMEA's income derived from an EU subsidy; by 2002, this proportion had fallen to about 14%, with most income derived from fees for the services that the agency provides. In 2002, the EMEA's budget was €70.5 million.

Document management and publishing

An electronic data management system has been introduced at the EMEA in which documents are held in a central location. They can then be circulated to all authorised recipients, and it can be assured that the latest version of the document is always in use.

There has also been a move towards the electronic submission of MAAs, with the electronic Common Technical Document project (eCTD) carried out under the auspices of the ICH process. eCTD defines a harmonised format (but not necessarily harmonised content) for submissions in the EU, the USA and Japan (see also Chapter 2).

A further initiative has been the product information management (PIM) project, jointly sponsored by the EMEA and EFPIA (European Federation of Pharmaceutical Industries and Associations). It is intended to define an exchange standard for product information used in SPCs, patient information and product packaging, and to facilitate the exchange of information between regulatory authorities and companies.

Meeting management and conferences

A considerable amount of time and resources is expended on meetings within the EMEA. In 2001, there were more than 320 meetings, with over 500 meeting days. Just over 3500 delegates were reimbursed for their attendance at meetings. To co-ordinate these activities, the agency utilises a computerised meeting management system, which was introduced in November 2001. Videoconferencing and teleconferencing facilities are also extensively used to try to reduce the costs of contacts with partners in other organisations.

Information technology (IT)

Extensive IT facilities are required to provide technology facilities and services for the smooth operation of the EMEA itself, and to support EU initiatives and activities. Two recent major projects have been the development of the EudraVigilance system for pharmacovigilance and the electronic document management system. A drugs approvals tracking system (SIAMED) has also been developed in collaboration with WHO.

Activities undertaken in support of European initiatives include the development of pan-European databases and electronic submission of data. It is also important that all competent authorities in the EU have access to the information held at the EMEA.

References

1. Council Directive 65/65/EEC of 26 January 1965 on the approximation of provisions laid down by law regulation or administrative action relating to medicinal products. *Official Journal of the European Communities* 1965; **P022**: 369.
2. Council Regulation (EEC) No. 2309/93 as amended, laying down Community procedures for the authorisation and supervision of medicinal products for human and veterinary use and establishing the EMEA. *Official Journal of the European Communities* 1993: **L214**: 1.

12

The National Institute for Clinical Excellence

The fundamental philosophy behind the assessment procedure carried out by a regulatory authority is that it is the quality, safety and efficacy of a medicinal product and the quality, safety and performance of a medical device that is considered. No judgement is made concerning the cost of the product or its relationship to other products within the same category of product (sometimes referred to as a 'fourth hurdle').

However, in view of the ever-increasing cost of healthcare budgets, most governments have now introduced some form of assessment of these latter two criteria. Such assessments are invariably kept separate from that carried out by the regulatory authority. The agency tasked with this in the UK is the National Institute for Clinical Excellence (NICE), a Special Health Authority, created in April 1999.

Objectives of NICE

NICE was established to provide clinical guidance and guidance on the clinical effectiveness and cost-effectiveness of new and existing clinical interventions to the National Health Service (NHS) in England and Wales. Proposals for setting up NICE were first described in the government's White Paper: *The New NHS: Modern and Dependable*, and further developed in the consultation paper *A First Class Service: Quality in the New NHS* and a follow-up discussion paper, *Faster Access to Modern Treatment: How NICE Appraisal Will Work*.

The fundamental objective is to improve standards of patient care, and to reduce inequities in access to innovative treatment, by establishing a process which:

- identifies new treatments and products which are likely to have a significant impact on the NHS, or which for other reasons would benefit from the issue of national guidance at an early stage
- enables evidence of clinical effectiveness and cost-effectiveness to be brought together to inform a judgement on the value of the treatment relative to alternative uses of resources in the NHS
- results in the issue of guidance on whether the treatment can be recommended for routine use in the NHS (and if so under what

conditions or for which groups of patients) together with a summary of the evidence on which the recommendation is based
- avoids any significant delays to those sponsoring the innovation either in meeting any national or international regulatory requirements or in bringing the innovation to market in the UK.

NICE is intended to appraise 30–50 new and existing interventions each year and issue guidance which aims:

- To promote the faster uptake of effective new treatments.
- To provide doctors with more support than previously in making complex decisions about individual patient care. It is recognised that there will be circumstances in which clinicians need to modify general guidance to fit individual patient circumstances. Overall, however, it is expected that NICE guidance will lead to greater equity of access to effective treatments across the NHS. Steps will be taken to ensure that variations in patient care which cannot be justified by genuine local differences are not allowed to persist.
- To enable the NHS to secure more health gain from available resources by focusing on treatments with clear evidence of cost-effectiveness.

The results of NICE's deliberations and its recommendations are sent to clinical professionals and commissioners in health authorities and primary care trusts. It also develops guidance for patients and carers on the implications for them of its recommendations.

Timely guidance is deemed necessary on individual treatments and products, and in particular clinical innovations. Frequently, when new treatments are introduced into general NHS practice, evidence of clinical effectiveness and cost-effectiveness is unclear or incomplete. This can cause:

- slow uptake, even of innovations of significant benefit
- different judgements across the country on the interpretation or significance of the evidence, resulting in variations in access for patients to the new treatments and the widespread perception of inequity
- wasteful use of resources as treatments are used outside the range of circumstances in which they are clinically effective and cost-effective, at the expense of alternative uses of those resources which could give greater benefits to patients.

In theory, it was considered beneficial to review all kinds of clinical intervention on an equal basis. This included:

- all therapeutic products, including medicines and medical devices
- all therapeutic interventions and programmes of care
- products and processes to diagnose and prevent disease
- population screening procedures.

However, priorities were set for the work programme, and consideration was made of how different health sectors (e.g. the medical device industry) can respond to the programme. Other sectors may already have effective arrangements in place (for example, population screening is covered by the work of the National Screening Committee).

Promotion of clinical effectiveness and cost-effectiveness

NICE promotes clinical effectiveness and cost-effectiveness by providing guidance and audit, in support of staff dealing with patients. It advises on best practice in using existing treatment options, appraising new health interventions, and advising the NHS on how they can be implemented and how best these might fit alongside existing treatments.

Dissemination of information

NICE also has a key role in coordinating the range of current activity both in the active dissemination of information and in responding to specific inquiries. It provides a single reference point for information on standards and audit methodologies, and supports and complements the new NHS Information Strategy (intended to provide universal desktop access to NICE guidance, along the lines of the PRODIGY computer-aided, decision-support system for general practitioners).

Implementation methodologies

NICE has developed a role in providing information about implementation methodologies to help local clinical teams. It has also ensured that its clinical guidance is integrated into other appropriate activities (e.g. professional education and training, seminars and workshops, patient education and information, and audit).

A new partnership

NICE has created a new partnership between the government, the NHS and clinical professionals. Through NICE, the government objective is to help clarify, for patients and professionals, which treatments work best for which patients and those which do not. The government, working with clinical bodies, systematically appraises clinical interventions before their introduction into the NHS. Thus, NICE gives doctors, nurses and midwives more support than previously available to facilitate their making the complex decisions about individual patient care. It also assists in the decisions made by those commissioning care.

Network of relationships

In support of its work, NICE has developed a network of relationships:

- Locally: with NHS Trusts, with other service providers, and with patient representatives to ensure that dissemination of guidance is

effective. It will also work with health authorities, primary care groups (local health groups in Wales) and other service commissioners.
- Regionally: receiving feedback from performance monitoring, addressing gaps in guidance and supporting local implementation.
- Nationally: organising a detailed work programme with the Department of Health and the National Assembly for Wales; working with Royal Colleges, professional associations, academic units and healthcare industries that have the specialist expertise required; and ensuring that information from the Commission for Health Improvement's systematic service reviews is fed into further clinical guidance or audit methodologies.

Other responsibilities

NICE has also taken over the funding, commissioning and oversight of a range of functions currently undertaken by a number of different groups funded by the Department of Health and the National Assembly for Wales. These functions include:

- the National Prescribing Centre appraisals and bulletins
- the clinical guidance contained in PRODIGY
- the National Centre for Clinical Audit
- the *Prescriber's Journal*
- the Department of Health-funded National Guidelines Programme and Professional Audit Programme
- Effectiveness Bulletins.

The Special Health Authority structure

The functions of NICE apply to the NHS in England and Wales. NICE was set up as a Special Health Authority in April 1999 (following the Establishment Order laid before Parliament on 2 January 1999) and is accountable to the Secretary of State for Health in England and the National Assembly for Wales for its resources, for delivery of its work programme and for the guidance it produces for the NHS. NICE is funded out of the money currently being spent on similar organisations and activities to those whose roles it will take on. Its annual budget on its establishment was about £9.8 million.

Executive Board

The Executive Board reflects a range of expertise, including the clinical professions, patients and user groups, NHS managers and research bodies. Members are appointed on merit, not as representatives of a particular organisation or interest. As a small body of executives and non-executives, the board ensures that NICE conducts its business on behalf of the NHS in the most effective way. The chief executive is accountable to the board for progress on the agreed programme and the use of resources.

Although NICE's executive board is not involved in the detail of each individual appraisal, it gives final authorisation for the issue of all guidance prepared by the appraisal group and directs the work of the appraisal group to ensure consistency with NICE's other work.

In addition, the board has to decide how best to handle cases in which sponsoring companies feel that the process operated by the appraisal group has not allowed them the to put their evidence in full.

Appraisal group

The appraisal group (see Table 12.1) is a subcommittee of NICE's executive board. Therefore, the chairperson of the group is accountable on all matters of policy and professional judgement to the chair of NICE. The head of the Secretariat is also accountable to NICE's chief executive for the performance of the appraisal group. All appraisal group advice is channelled through NICE and is issued with NICE's authority. Additional ad hoc members may be appointed by the chair, the vice-chair or the chief executive.

The appraisal group also (through the Secretariat) has access to a wide range of subject specialists. These specialists are invited to comment, usually in writing, but also at the committee's deliberations if required. They do not contribute to the appraisal group's final decisions, but advise on specialist aspects of procedures under discussion.

Partners' Council

The NICE Partners' Council comprises representatives of all the key stakeholder groups (patients and carers, the health professions including the

Table 12.1 Professional membership of the Appraisal Group

Chair	× 1
Hospital physicians	× 2
Pharmaceutical physician	× 1
Surgeon	× 1
Diagnostic pathologist	× 1
General practitioners	× 2
Public health physician	× 1
Hospital nurse	× 1
Community nurse	× 1
Health economists	× 3
Pharmacist	× 1
Biostatistician	× 1
Patient advocates	× 2
Health managers	× 3

professional Royal Colleges, academics, NHS service interests and the pharmaceutical and other healthcare industries). The council is appointed by the Secretaries of State for Health and for Wales. Its role includes reviewing NICE's annual progress report and contributing to the development of the work programme, commissioned by the Department of Health and Welsh Office.

Secretariat

The NICE Secretariat initially consisted of staff from the Department of Health who provided technical and administrative support. It also has professional, academic and managerial skills to commission and manage the guidance and audit programmes and to support the national appraisal function. The Secretariat has a wider role in the coordination of NICE's work programme across a range of organisations.

The Secretariat prepares initial evaluations of evidence for the appraisal group, to allow discussion to focus on key issues. The Secretariat also assists in drafting the appraisal group's recommendations and in handling enquiries about its work, both generally and in individual cases. The Secretariat comprises the following expertise:

- clinical epidemiology
- health economics
- statistical analysis
- research methodology
- literature search and library skills
- drafting of clinical guidance.

Memorandum of understanding on appraisal of health interventions

A Memorandum of Understanding (MOU) on appraisal of health interventions sets out the rules under which NICE carries out its appraisals. Appraisals are intended to promote the appropriate use of interventions which offer good value to patients and to discourage the use of those which do not. It builds on the proposals set out in the discussion paper *A First Class Service: Quality in the New NHS*, modified in the light of comments received and further discussion with stakeholders.

Selection of topics – horizon scanning

The responsibility for selection of topics to be referred to NICE lies with the Department of Health, in consultation with the National Assembly for Wales, NICE and other interested parties. In practice, new interventions are selected from those innovations which are deemed likely to have significant impact on the NHS. This appraisal is carried out on behalf of the Department of Health by the National Horizon Scanning Centre at the University of Birmingham. Selection criteria include topics covered by National Service Frameworks or those where there is widespread variation in clinical practice or uncertainty over best practice.

The Department of Health gives final notification of referral of interventions to NICE no later than 9 months before the point at which guidance is to be ready for dissemination. Exceptionally, a shorter notice period may be necessary (e.g. when a technology is changing rapidly or when new evidence radically alters the perception of an existing technology).

The National Horizon Scanning Centre and the National Prescribing Centre for medicines have been commissioned to carry out horizon scanning on behalf of the NHS Executive. To do this, they scan published material, maintain contacts with similar groups in other countries, and establish informal contacts with clinicians and researchers, patient groups, sponsoring companies and industry associations.

A standing 'short-list' is produced, summarising areas of application, possible benefits, and likely impact on NHS resources. For medicinal products under development, bulletins based on these summaries are published by the National Prescribing Centre/Drug Information Pharmacists Group about 6–12 months before the medicinal product is expected to receive a marketing authorisation.

The Department of Health regularly and systematically examines all the interventions on the short-list, focusing in particular on those expected to be launched in about 6 years' time or less. Where an intervention will probably be selected for appraisal, the Department will notify the sponsoring company and invite comments. The judgement that a particular intervention is likely to qualify for appraisal will be reviewed annually, and the sponsoring company notified of any changes. The Department notifies NICE of its provisional judgements to enable forward planning of the programme of appraisals.

If there is no obvious sponsoring company, the Department decides whether any research should be commissioned through the NHS R&D programme.

When an intervention has been provisionally selected for appraisal, and it is likely to be marketed to the NHS within the subsequent 12 months, the Department finalises its selection decision and gives the sponsoring company a final opportunity to make representations. Subject to this:

- The company is formally notified that an appraisal will be needed and is invited to submit evidence by, generally, no later than 4 months before the intended launch, or, in the case of pharmaceuticals, the time of submission to the regulatory authorities.
- Similarly any relevant patient groups are invited to submit any views by the same deadline.
- NICE is formally invited to carry out the appraisal.

Work programme

Initial work programme

NICE published in August 1999 the initial batch of technologies that ministers wished it to start appraising in autumn 1999. It wrote to the following, inviting them to submit evidence for the appraisal:

- manufacturers of the technologies
- 'appropriate' NHS groups
- professional organisations
- patient groups with an interest.

The list of interventions for the initial work programme is given in Table 12.2.

Future work programme

The Department of Health regularly determines the future work programme for NICE, and those technologies it is required to consider each year.

The appraisal process

General issues

The appraisal process used by NICE was set out in a Memorandum of Understanding, published in August 1999 (see page 200) and in *Appraisal of New and Existing Technologies: Interim Guidance for Manufacturers and Sponsors*. The memorandum outlined arrangements for submitting evidence, consulting on draft guidance, and instigating appeals in the event of dispute over final recommendations from NICE.

It is intended that the appraisal process will have no effect on requirements for medicinal products obtaining a marketing authorisation or on safety requirements for medical devices (determined by the application of a CE mark). The process is formally independent of the processes operated in each case by the UK Medicines and Healthcare products Regulatory Agency (MHRA).

Detailed methodology has been developed for judging the evidence and reaching an overall view on the clinical effectiveness and cost-effectiveness of the intervention. The appraisal considers some or all of the following points:

- How robust is the assessment? For example, if the assessment used modelling (e.g. to get from measurable clinical outcomes to impact on quality of life), are the assumptions clinically credible? Evidence is required on clinical outcomes relative to no treatment and/or best

Table 12.2 Initial NICE work programme

Treatment	Notes
Hip prostheses/hip replacement	There was no evidence of additional benefit from using more expensive prostheses from two recent studies in the NHS health technology assessment (HTA) programme. NICE will examine this and other evidence and produce an assessment of the issue. NICE will also advise how the NHS could obtain best value-for-money without reducing quality of patient care.
Advances in hearing aids/ hearing disability	There have been significant recent developments in hearing aid technology, but provision both of new and conventional aids is variable. Guidance from NICE will establish basic standards, and may assess any additional benefits from newer aids.
Routine extraction of wisdom teeth/dental care	Professional opinion is increasingly stating that routine extraction of nonsymptomatic wisdom teeth is unnecessary (and some related procedures involve the risk of actual harm). This is supported by guidelines from the Faculty of Dental Surgery and from the Scottish Inter-Collegiate Network, and by a critical review from York University. Nevertheless, a significant number of dentists continue to carry this out. Guidance from NICE will give clear standards, possibly leading to the phasing out of many unnecessary and potentially harmful treatments.
Liquid-based cytology/ cervical screening	This is one of a number of current developments in screening technology, and the one most likely to have early impact on the NHS. This technique should improve the quality and readability of slides, thus reducing the number of false negatives. Its use, however, involves significant capital investment, a major reorganisation of the service and a significant increase in running costs. NICE will consider the evidence and advise whether this technology offers worthwhile benefits.
Coronary artery stent developments/treatment of coronary heart disease	Stent insertion, to reduce the risk of coronary arteries blocking up again after angioplasty, is very common. However, there are doubts over its appropriate use, especially in view of the variations to the basic technique being developed. NICE has been asked to survey these developments as well as the underlying case for using stent technology.
Taxanes: paclitaxel (Taxol) ovarian cancer, breast cancer; docetaxel (Taxotere) breast cancer	The taxanes are existing drugs with well-established uses in treatment of a range of cancers. The current uncertainty concerns the use of paclitaxel as a first-line treatment in ovarian cancer. Both drugs may be newly indicated in the treatment of advanced breast cancer. Because of their relatively high cost and some difficulties over interpreting the clinical evidence, NICE will give definitive advice on the available evidence.
Inhaler systems (devices) for childhood asthma	A wide range of devices have been developed to enable patients to inhale effective doses of anti-asthma drugs. There is much debate over the clinical effectiveness and cost-effectiveness of more sophisticated systems, and therefore much variation in practice. The issues are particularly problematic in very young children (up to 5 years) who may have difficulty in using simpler, cheaper devices.

continued

Table 12.2 Initial NICE work programme (*cont.*)

Treatment	Notes
Proton pump inhibitors (PPIs) for treatment of dyspepsia	PPIs are very clinically effective and cost-effective for some patients, but there is good evidence of their inappropriate use in two instances: treatment of minor disease which would have responded to less expensive treatments; and failure to attack the underlying cause of ulcers by using *H. pylori* eradication therapy after initial treatment of symptoms with a PPI. Clear guidance from NICE offers the potential for significant savings while enhancing quality of care.
Interferon beta (relapsing remitting/secondary progressive MS); glatiramer (relapsing remitting MS)	Interferon beta is a controversial treatment for patients with a poor prognosis and no effective alternative, and upon which high patient hopes have developed. Many clinicians have major doubts over the cost-effectiveness of this treatment and the scope for successful targeting of patients most likely to benefit.
	On the available evidence, the new product glatiramer (expected to receive a marketing authorisation imminently) will raise similar issues. It is proposed that NICE should consider pharmaceutical treatment in the context of services for MS patients generally; NICE may subsequently be asked to follow up this appraisal of the role of the two pharmaceuticals by developing a more wide-ranging guideline to set standards for care in MS.
Zanamivir/oseltamivir for influenza	Evidence suggests these two new drugs can shorten the duration of influenza by up to 2 days if taken soon after symptoms appear. Effective use will depend critically on how successfully they could be targeted at those most likely to benefit, without increasing the pressure on primary care services at what is already a difficult time of year. NICE guidance could help set the evidence of clinical benefit in its proper context, including the appropriate use of preventative measures such as vaccination.

existing treatment for the condition in question, including undesirable side-effects and (for chronic conditions) effects of stopping treatment.
- What is the estimated impact on quality and (where appropriate) length of life?
- What is the estimated average health improvement per treatment initiated, expressed as standard measures for combining life years and quality of life?
- For factors which can be quantified, is there convincing evidence that the proposed intervention is likely to be cost-effective, on the basis of the health improvement achieved for given NHS resources, compared with other potential uses of those resources?
- How far is clinical effectiveness and cost-effectiveness affected when other health-related costs and benefits are taken into account (where relevant)?
- What factors should be considered which cannot be quantified, but are still relevant to assessing clinical effectiveness and cost-effectiveness?

- Taking all factors into account, can the treatment be recommended as generally clinically effective and cost-effective?
- Are there any particular subgroups for which the treatment is likely to be more or less clinically effective and cost-effective? Should treatment be targeted on the groups who would derive most benefit?
- Should use of the intervention be subject to particular conditions (e.g. skills/training of the clinicians who initiate/continue treatment, requirements for monitoring/review, quality control, indications for stopping treatment)?
- What factors should be discussed between clinician and patient for an informed joint decision to be made in individual cases (e.g. overall balance of risks and benefits, rare side-effects, alternative treatments)?
- What is the total likely impact on NHS resources (including manpower resources) and, where different, on government funding of health care as a whole? What are the net NHS costs associated with this health gain?
- Are there (where appropriate) any associated government-funded Personal Social Services costs and savings?
- In the light of the group's discussions, what further research would be desirable either (a) to put the conclusions on a firmer basis or (b) to indicate how the intervention should best be used?
- Are there other issues not detected by the above steps which are relevant to the appraisal?

Submission of evidence

Evidence submitted is appraised by NICE in consultation with interested parties. NICE has the objective of applying equal rigour to its appraisal of all types of intervention.

Data/evidence required from a single sponsoring company

The data submitted by a sponsoring company is analysed, and the company is contacted to clarify points. The Secretariat appends a commentary to the data which reviews the robustness of the evidence submitted, and adds to the analysis as needed (e.g. supplying an analysis of the impact on NHS resources if the sponsoring company has not included this in the submission).

The commentary is sent to the sponsoring company, who can add comments. Comments are also invited from any relevant patient groups, either on their own initiative or in response to the industry submission and/or secretariat comments. The Department of Health, National Assembly for Wales or NHS bodies (e.g. the NHS Confederation) are also invited to submit views.

When the process is complete, the full set of papers (containing the sponsoring company's submission, any other initial submissions, Secretariat commentary, and further comments from the company and other interested parties) are given to the appraisal group.

Data/evidence required when there is no sponsoring company

If there is no sponsoring company (e.g. as for most surgical procedures), NICE invites the Department of Health to commission an assessment. This typically is from academic groups (e.g. those who already have experience of similar work on behalf of the regional Development Evaluation Committees (DECs)). The assessment reviews existing and/or new research as appropriate. Patient groups are also invited to submit views. The process then continues as above.

Data/evidence required from several sponsors

If there are a number of alternative devices for a single procedure, or there are a number of alternative treatments (none of which has been previously appraised), more than one sponsor may be involved.

To deal with this situation, the Department can commission research on the clinical effectiveness of the procedure in generic terms. This considers variations associated with particular products, drawing as far as possible on research already carried out by individual sponsoring companies. Combined with information on the cost of individual products, this creates an assessment of the relative clinical effectiveness and cost-effectiveness of each product. The submission to NICE is made by the group carrying out the research, but each company (and relevant patient groups) can add comments on the overall assessment or on aspects relating to its individual product.

Confidentiality issues

NICE bears in mind very carefully issues of confidentiality. Ideally, NICE's processes should be as transparent as possible and the evidence underlying its recommendations should be accessible. However, NICE recognises that, to operate effectively, it has to be supplied with information from sponsors that is not in the public domain at the time of appraisal. In many cases, this information will be commercially confidential. Sponsors are reluctant to make it available unless they are assured that it will not be disclosed outside NICE.

NICE has adopted policies which reflect these objectives. They take into account current legal requirements (including any future freedom of information legislation) and prevailing understandings between government, industry and the general public on information in regulatory submissions.

Review of the initial appraisal

The initial appraisal and guidance from NICE can be subjected to review when limited approval is given to a health intervention, allowing further research or development. Subsequently, the sponsoring company is invited to make a further submission, describing how its new data amend the original decision.

Review may also be necessary when further information on benefits or costs (e.g. concerning either an intervention or comparison treatments) becomes available which changes the basis of a previous appraisal. The additional data may come from the appraisal Secretariat, from an individual member of the appraisal group, or from the sponsoring company. The appraisal group considers whether to review its earlier guidance. If necessary, it invites the sponsoring company to make a full submission.

Timescale

The appraisal process should not delay the introduction of innovations into clinical practice. Indeed, appraisals sometimes expedite the use of beneficial new interventions throughout the NHS. The process described in *Appraisal of New and Existing Technologies: Interim Guidance for Manufacturers and Sponsors* suggested an overall timetable of up to 8 months from submission of evidence to issue of guidance. Additional time can be allowed at the sponsor company's request if the company wishes to submit further evidence in the light of the Secretariat's commentary.

The appraisal period incorporates time for the sponsoring company, patient groups, the Department of Health and the National Assembly for Wales to receive the draft recommendations and make final comments. The appraisal group reviews its recommendations before they are issued in their final form.

Application to existing interventions

In both the cases described below, the appraisal process is essentially the same as for new interventions. However, the appraisal group also has to consider those patients who are established on treatments subsequently shown not to meet the criteria of clinical effectiveness and cost-effectiveness. The group advises on when clinicians should be encouraged to attempt to switch such patients to alternatives. There are two elements to the 'catch-up' programme for existing health interventions.

Assessments completed under the Department of Health's Health Technology Assessment (HTA) Programme

Upon completion of each HTA assessment, the Department of Health uses the same selection criteria as those for new interventions. Interventions meeting the criteria are automatically referred to the appraisal group, with the HTA assessment forming the central platform of evidence (supplemented as required by further analysis, commissioned from the original research group or from one of the regular assessment providers). The Department ensures that this does not inadvertently give a competitive advantage to one product, although application of the suggested selection criteria normally avoids this.

Systematic prioritised catch-up programme

Over several years, the Department has prioritised the most significant existing interventions for appraisal, using a modified version of the selection criteria. Interventions were more likely to be selected if there was evidence of significant variations in NHS use, or of use not in accordance with generally accepted Good Clinical Practice. Where necessary, the department has commissioned an assessment of the selected intervention through the NHS R&D programme.

Guidance documents

The guidance documents form the crux of the output from NICE. They include the primary appraisal assessment, giving NICE's guidance on when an intervention is recommended for routine NHS clinical use.

Format and content of NICE's guidance

If the advice is to succeed in enhancing resource use and reducing disparities in the uptake of the intervention, the recommendations must be clear and precise. The recommendations are expressed as a limited number of categories:

A   Recommended as clinically effective and cost-effective for routine NHS use (for all indications, for specific indications, and/or only for particular patient subgroups). This is further qualified as recommended for use by all GPs and specialists, in hospitals and for GPs with particular expertise (and agreed by joint formulary or shared care arrangements), or only in specialist (tertiary referral) centres.

B   Recommended only for use in clinical trials set up to research cost-effectiveness and targeting.

C   Not recommended for routine use.

NICE's advice can also incorporate indications for use, training, issues to be raised with patients in seeking informed consent, monitoring and evaluation, indications for stopping treatment, any priorities for treatment, and an assessment of any wider implications for the NHS. A summary of the evidence on which the appraisal is based, giving the reasoning behind NICE's recommendations, forms part of the guidance. As far as practicable, all evidence sources are made available for inspection.

Legal status of guidance

All guidance is fully reasoned and written in terms which make clear that it is guidance. Guidance for clinicians does not override their professional responsibility to make an appropriate decision in an individual's circumstances, in consultation with the patient or guardian/carer and in the light of any locally agreed policies. Similarly, guidance to NHS trusts and commissioners does not take away their discretion under administrative law to take account of individual circumstances.

Implications for guidelines and other information

Where appropriate, NICE ensures that the implications of its recommendations are carried through to:

- related clinical guidelines
- PRODIGY guidelines
- the National Electronic Library for Health
- the protocols used by NHS Direct and NHS Walk-in Centres, and any material for patients produced by NHS Direct Online.

The guidance from the appraisal process is different in nature and purpose from clinical guidelines. To prevent confusion, however, NICE ensures that the appraisal group has considered any guidelines relevant to the intervention they are appraising. Conversely, any future clinical guideline development must incorporate the results of NICE appraisals of any relevant interventions.

This is facilitated by regular liaison between the respective Secretariats, some common membership of the appraisal group and the professional advisory group overseeing NICE's guidelines programme, and overview of the final outcomes by the NICE board. The same principles apply to the relation between the appraisal process and the department's initiative on computerised decision support (PRODIGY).

Dissemination of information to patients and carers

Patients and carers have a right to information on their condition and its treatment so that they can discuss treatment choices on an informed basis with their clinicians. This information needs to be unbiased, authoritative and intelligible. Patients and carers also have a right to information on the basis of recommendations adopted by NICE which affect the available treatment options. To achieve this, NICE has consulted with appropriate patient groups and bodies such as the Centre for Health Information on the best format and means of dissemination. This guidance *inter alia* explains the nature of the clinical recommendations, the implications for the standards which patients can expect, and the broad nature of the evidence on which the recommendations are based.

Appraisal process in the event of an uncertain outcome

It is possible that the appraisal group may decide that a proposed intervention is potentially of value but that there is insufficient evidence to justify an unqualified positive recommendation by NICE. This was most likely to arise during the 3-year maturation period. To deal with this, NICE can:

- recommend further research to see whether the potential promise of the intervention can be realised
- specify the issues which this research should address
- advise that, in the meantime, clinicians should only use the new intervention as part of a well-designed programme of clinical research directed at these questions.

Exceptionally, and during the maturation period only – and where uncertainty relates only to details of clinical practice, not to the assessment of clinical effectiveness and cost-effectiveness – NICE may recommend wider adoption of the treatment, as long as the necessary research is to be carried out.

Sponsoring companies fund further research advised by NICE. They are also encouraged to discuss with the Department of Health's R&D Directorate the best way of organising this research. If there is no sponsoring company for a particular intervention, the Department of Health considers whether it should fund the required research.

Transitional arrangements

Transitional arrangements were needed. For medicinal products, any clinical research needed to satisfy requirements to obtain a marketing authorisation was already under way. It was therefore unreasonable to require information which was not obtainable from this research, since additional research might delay product launch.

The medical device industry faced different problems. Current European legislation (Directive 90/342/EEC, which covers about 90% of all medical devices) requires evidence only of quality and safety, not of clinical efficacy (all three are required for medicinal products). Assessment of clinical effectiveness and cost-effectiveness is not easy or cheap. Some of the smaller medical devices companies found it difficult to fund clinical trials to produce evidence of clinical effectiveness and cost-effectiveness. It was also much more likely that a number of medical device companies would be developing similar products for the same procedure. In recognition of this, it was planned that:

- The information requirements which applied when the system was mature would be published at the earliest opportunity.
- Sponsoring companies would be invited to approach the Secretariat at the earliest possible stage – especially for interventions on the department's provisional short list of candidates for appraisal – and discuss what clinical research (if any) was already in train,

and whether it would be possible to modify or extend it to provide information which would not be a direct output of the research.
- The Secretariat would be given the discretion to agree that, where it would be unreasonable or disproportionately expensive to expect the sponsoring company to provide research evidence fully conforming to the requirements, any 'gaps' can be filled by modelling. The Secretariat also had the discretion to discuss information gaps with the Department, who in exceptional cases could agree to commission research to help fill the gaps. The sponsoring company might be required to make a contribution to the cost.
- In such cases the sponsoring company had to indicate, as part of their submission, what further post-marketing research it intended to carry out to fill any remaining gaps in the available evidence.

Proposed data requirements for sponsors' submissions

A standard reporting format assists preparation of submissions by the Secretariat of the appraisal group. It acts as a checklist, ensuring that essential information is not omitted and helping organisation of the work involved in producing the submission and in appraising its contents.

Summary and introductory remarks

Sponsors must provide an executive summary. It compares results to alternative therapies and describes limitations of the analysis, and makes appropriate recommendations for NHS use.

An introduction to the main submission follows the summary. It should describe the disease, its epidemiology, current practice, and the significance in terms of ill health and resource costs of treating it. It should describe the intervention being assessed and the indications for which a recommendation is sought. For medicinal products, the description should include therapeutic classification, brand and generic name, dosage form and route, and all indications for which a marketing authorisation is being sought or has been obtained. Specific patient subgroups to which the analysis is being applied should be defined.

Sponsors have to disclose their relationship with the author of the study. It should be clear how much of the submission the author agrees with, and to what extent the author is independent of the sponsor.

Methods

Study design

The submission should specify whether the study design was prospective, retrospective, modelled or a mixture. The analytical framework and reasons for adopting the study design should be set out. Departures from incremental cost–utility analysis should be justified.

Timescale

The choice of timescale of the assessment should also be justified, by showing that significant costs or benefits beyond the chosen horizon are unlikely.

Related and comparative studies

All related studies of the therapy and its comparators (and especially all randomised clinical trials) should be reviewed and fully referenced. If the results of any of these are excluded from the analysis, reasons should be fully given.

The choice of comparator therapy should be explained and any reasons for not following guideline recommendations. The method adopted for comparing clinical efficacy should be given (e.g. randomised control trial, meta-analysis, or other specified methods).

Outcome measurement

The approach used should be detailed. All outcome variables considered should be mentioned. Reasons should be given for rejecting any outcomes considered and for ignoring any outcomes actually measured. For all outcomes included, the method of measurement should be given. The methods, evidence base and assumptions used in deriving clinical efficacy results should be described. Other clinical and sociodemographic data collected in trials should also be listed.

Methods used to assess quality of life

These should be described and justified where quality of life is a significant factor in the assessment. If an attempt has been made to measure quality of life directly, the focus will be on the performance of the measuring instrument. When quality of life is modelled indirectly from clinical endpoints, it will be more important to demonstrate the evidence underpinning the modelling.

Costs

It should be clear how costs have been estimated and who bears them. The sources should be given for both resource use and price data, and assumptions should be stated explicitly.

Uncertainty

Major sources of uncertainty should be highlighted. Do they arise from sampling error or from the range of plausible assumptions? Any major assumptions and limitations contained in the analysis should also be highlighted.

Results – outcomes

The analysis should be reported step by step, proceeding from the base data through any systematic review, meta-analysis and modelling, to final estimates of efficacy and effectiveness relative to comparator therapy. The structure for reporting should therefore be:

- results of individual trials or observational studies
- results of reviews and meta-analysis
- modelled results (showing how derived)
- overall conclusions on efficacy and effectiveness, including estimated increase in health gain relative to the comparator.

The level of detail required is the minimum necessary to enable replication of the results from base data. Additional data may, however, be requested.

Results – costs related to health treatment

Sufficient information should be given to enable sources of all cost estimates to be traced. The following items should be separately identified:

- costs to the NHS
- health-related costs to the government-funded Personal Social Services, where relevant
- costs avoided as a result of the therapy, classified as beneficiary
- capital and overhead costs
- costs arising in different years (with and without discounting).

A wider range of costs and benefits may be relevant in particular cases. The Secretariat has advised in individual cases how costs and benefits arising outside the NHS should be handled.

Results – sensitivity and subgroups

Sources of uncertainty not deriving from sampling error should be presented in a sensitivity analysis. A decision tree should be considered where there are several important sources of uncertainty.

Cost-effectiveness results for each identified subgroup should be set out, identifying any economically significant differences.

Aggregate cost impacts

The submission should estimate the number of patients for whom the therapy is likely to be clinically effective and cost-effective, and derive from this an estimate of the total cost to the NHS of adopting it. A profile of costs over time should be given. A sensitivity analysis should show how these estimates are affected by extending treatment to all patients with indications for which the therapy has, or will have, regulatory approval.

Equity issues

The sociodemographic characteristics of the beneficiaries should be noted where they are a nonrepresentative sample of the UK population. It is important to highlight treatments which could have a significant impact on health inequalities by gender, ethnic group or socioeconomic category, or on a group particularly disadvantaged owing to the nature of their disease.

Other unquantifiable factors

Any other unquantifiable factors should be described. These include factors which cannot be reflected in quantified assessment of health gain but which the sponsoring company believes are relevant to the final assessment of clinical effectiveness and cost-effectiveness. Any relevant details should also be given which would help the appraisal group judge their significance. The appraisal group might issue further guidance at a later stage on the factors which are likely to be relevant.

Conclusions

The final part of the submission should draw together the main results, assumptions, limitations and uncertainties. These should be in the context of relevant alternative therapies and present a reasoned conclusion based on the estimated increase in health gain and any other relevant factors.

13

International perspectives

Although this book has concentrated largely upon the regulatory environment in the UK, it is evident that the UK cannot and does not operate in isolation in the regulation of medicines and medical devices. Indeed, as shown in Chapter 1, the involvement of Europe, especially in the control of medicinal products, began almost 40 years ago and has continued apace since then.

The cost of developing new medicinal products and medical devices has also had a significant bearing on the structure and functioning of the pharmaceutical industry. Globalisation of many of its activities, with multiple mergers creating supranational organisations, has led to a relatively small number of very large pharmaceutical companies, many of whom are based in the USA but with offices spread throughout the world.

This chapter considers the processes by which regulatory authorities and pharmaceutical companies have reacted to these changes. It reviews the ways in which the requirements for registration of medicinal products have begun to be harmonised across the globe; the role of the US Food and Drug Administration (FDA), the largest regulatory authority in the world; and (briefly) the role of the World Health Organization (WHO) in the regulation of medicinal products.

Global harmonisation – the ICH process

Part A of this book makes clear the volume and complexity of the data that companies must submit to obtain a marketing authorisation. Almost all countries have at least one regulatory authority dealing with medicinal products. Sometimes the authority deals with human medicinal products, veterinary medicinal products and medical devices. Alternatively, there may be separate authorities for each of these types of product.

The function of all regulatory authorities is to safeguard public (and animal) health; they must also ensure that new treatments are available to the benefit of patients at the earliest opportunity. Over time, each national regulatory authority has established national rules and regulations to control the development of new medicinal products and their use, and to monitor their performance after the marketing authorisation has been given. However, the piecemeal development of controls over time inevitably led to differing requirements in different countries. To maximise the return on their research and development costs, pharmaceutical companies usually seek to market their products in as many countries as possible. However, to do so, they have had to tailor the data submitted in support of a marketing authorisation application (MAA) for each country's differing demands.

Another aspect of this issue is that there is a great deal of duplication of the assessment work carried out by regulatory authorities. This leads to unnecessary costs diverted away from the overall health budget at a time when all countries are trying to ensure the most cost-effective use of limited resources.

This dual problem has been less pronounced in the EU since the introduction of Directive 65/65/EEC, although it has only been since the late 1980s that all EU Member States have followed essentially the same legislative requirements. Moreover, this has not eliminated the sometimes idiosyncratic interpretation of that legislation, especially that based on Directives, which have to be transposed into national legislation before they become legally binding.

Moreover, those countries that have applied to become and were integrated as full members of the EU in 2004 have had to demonstrate that they can adopt and implement current legislation in full as a prerequisite of EU membership. An ambitious programme, the Pan-European Regulatory Forum (PERF), has, since 1998, been instrumental in assisting new members to become fully integrated prior to their accession. The nine or ten new members, mainly from central and eastern Europe, were therefore able to operate in a way that was harmonised with the existing 15 Member States from day one.

Beyond the boundaries of the enlarged EU, however, the situation and requirements have developed very differently. From its inception, the US FDA adopted a more prescriptive attitude to pharmaceutical controls: the rules laid down in the Code of Federal Regulations (CFR) have to be followed to the letter. This is in direct contrast to the reliance on guidance alongside primary legislation adopted by the EU.

The third major market for pharmaceuticals, both in usage and in manufacture, is Japan. Until recently, it was very difficult for non-Japanese companies to be able to market their products in Japan. Over the past 15 years, however, the Japanese market has become much more open as Japan has embraced the trends towards global harmonisation of pharmaceutical controls.

Tackling the problem

The International Conference on Harmonisation of Technical Requirements for Registration of Pharmaceuticals for Human Use (ICH) was the tangible result of this desire for global efficiency in the control of medicinal products. Its inaugural international meeting was held in April 1990. It has held major conferences approximately every 2 years to formalise and publicise the work carried out in the period since the previous conference and to plan future topics to be covered. (A parallel process for the harmonisation of the regulation of veterinary medicinal products, VICH, was begun some 5 years later. There is also a Global Harmonisation Task Force (GHTF) for medical devices, which has similar objectives.)

What is ICH?

ICH is a process by which the regulatory authorities of the USA, the EU and Japan, and experts from pharmaceutical industry trade associations in the three regions, meet to try to agree common requirements for registration of medicinal products. The objective is to discuss scientific and technical aspects of medicinal product registration. The six founder members of the ICH Steering Committee are listed in Table 13.1; observers and the Secretariat are also detailed.

On the tenth anniversary of the ICH process in 2000, a set of revised Terms of Reference were published:

- To maintain a forum for a constructive dialogue between regulatory authorities and the pharmaceutical industry on the real and perceived differences in the technical requirements for product registration in the EU, the USA and Japan in order to ensure a more timely introduction of new medicinal products, and their availability to patients.
- To contribute to the protection of public health from an international perspective.
- To monitor and update harmonised technical requirements leading to a greater mutual acceptance of research and development data.
- To avoid divergent future requirements through harmonisation of selected topics needed as a result of therapeutic advances and the development of new technologies for the production of medicinal products.
- To facilitate the adoption of new or improved technical research and development approaches which update or replace current practices, where these permit a more economical use of human, animal and material resources, without compromising safety.
- To facilitate the dissemination and communication of information on harmonised guidelines and their use such as to encourage the implementation and integration of common standards.

ICH Co-ordinators

An ICH Co-ordinator is nominated by each of the six co-sponsors as the main point of contact with the ICH Secretariat. The Co-ordinator ensures that ICH documents are distributed to appropriate parties. A Contact Network of experts within each organisation or region is also set up by each co-sponsor. This helps ensure that the views and policies of the co-sponsor they represent are presented.

Table 13.1 Members of and observers to the ICH Steering Committee

The six co-sponsors are equal partners in the process and each has two seats on the ICH Steering Committee (SC) which oversees harmonisation activities. IFPMA provides the Secretariat and participates as a nonvoting member of the Steering Committee. The Observers nominate participants to attend the ICH Steering Committee Meetings

Europe

European Commission/European Union (EU)
The European Commission represents the EU Member States. The Commission is working, through harmonisation of technical requirements and procedures, to achieve a single market in pharmaceuticals which would allow free movement of products throughout the EU.

European Federation of Pharmaceutical Industries and Associations (EFPIA)
EFPIA is based in Brussels and its members are Member Associations of 16 Member States in western Europe. Much of the Federation's work is concerned with the activities of the European Commission and the EMEA.

EFPIA member companies are manufacturers of prescription medicines and include all of Europe's primary research-based pharmaceutical companies. To ensure that EFPIA's views expressed at ICH are representative of the industry, a network of experts and country co-ordinators has been established in Member Associations.

Japan

Ministry of Health, Labor, and Welfare, Japan (MHLW)
The statutory responsibilities of the MHLW are to improve and promote social welfare, social security and public health. The Pharmaceutical Affairs Bureau, which is one of nine MHLW Offices, contains the Pharmaceuticals and Cosmetics Division. The Division is responsible for reviewing data and licensing medicinal products and cosmetics; it also acts as the focus for ICH activities.

The National Institute of Health Sciences (NIHS) and academia carry out research and testing on drugs, vaccines and biologicals. Technical advice on ICH matters is obtained through MHLW's regulatory expert groups, which include members from NIHS.

Japan Pharmaceutical Manufacturers Association (JPMA)
JPMA represents 90 companies who include all the major research-based pharmaceutical manufacturers in Japan. ICH work is co-ordinated through committees of industry experts, who also participate in the ICH Expert Working Groups.

JPMA promotes the development of a competitive pharmaceutical industry by a greater awareness and understanding of international issues. It also promotes the adoption of international standards by its member companies.

USA

US Food and Drug Administration (FDA)
The US Food and Drug Administration has responsibilities for drugs, biologicals, medical devices, cosmetics and radiological products. It is the largest of the world's drug regulatory authorities.

FDA comprises administrative, scientific and regulatory staff. Technical advice and experts for ICH are drawn from the Center for Drug Evaluation and Research (CDER) and the Center for Biologics Evaluation and Research (CBER).

Pharmaceutical Research and Manufacturers of America (PhRMA)
The Pharmaceutical Research and Manufacturers of America represents 67 research-based companies in the USA and 24 research affiliates.

continued

Table 13.1 Members of and observers to the ICH Steering Committee (*cont.*)

PhRMA, previously known as the US Pharmaceutical Manufacturers Association (PMA), co-ordinates its technical input to ICH through its Scientific and Regulatory Section. Special expert committees deal with specific ICH topics.

Observers
The following observers act as a link with non-ICH countries and regions:

- The World Health Organisation (WHO)
- The European Free Trade Area (EFTA), represented at ICH by Switzerland
- Canada, represented at ICH by the Drugs Directorate, Health Canada

Each Observer has a seat on the ICH Steering Committee

Secretariat – IFPMA
The International Federation of Pharmaceutical Manufacturers Association (IFPMA) is a Federation of member associations which represents the research-based pharmaceutical industry and other manufacturers of prescription medicines in 56 countries globally. IFPMA ensures contact on ICH matters with the research-based industry outside ICH Regions. IFPMA has two seats on the ICH Steering Committee and runs the ICH Secretariat.

The ICH Secretariat

The Secretariat is based in IFPMA's offices in Geneva. Its primary function is the organisation of Steering Committee meetings and the associated documentation; it also organises Expert Working Group (EWG) meetings. The Secretariat organises the technical documentation and liaises with speakers.

Transparency of the ICH process

The title of the ICH process stemmed from the original intention to hold one or more international conferences on the harmonisation process. However, 'ICH' has now become synonymous with the harmonisation process, not just the conferences. Nevertheless, the conferences have provided an important showcase for the transparency of the harmonisation programme.

The inaugural meeting of the Steering Committee was held in Brussels in April 1990. Since then, major international meetings have taken place, usually every 2 years in each of the three regions (see Table 13.2). Organisation of a conference is dealt with by the industry and regulatory authority or authorities in whose country/region the conference is taking place.

Regional Workshops on implementing and using ICH guidelines have sometimes taken place alongside a Steering Committee meeting. Future workshops are likely and will provide a forum for wider discussion of the guidelines and their implementation.

Table 13.2 Major ICH conferences

Date	Conference	Location
November 2003	ICH 6	Osaka, Japan
November 2000	ICH 5	San Diego, USA
July 1997	ICH 4	Brussels, Belgium
November 1995	ICH 3	Yokohama, Japan
October 1993	ICH 2	Orlando, USA
November 1991	ICH 1	Brussels, Belgium

ICH Expert Working Groups (EWGs)

The work of the ICH is carried out by Expert Working Groups (EWGs). The ICH Steering Committee appoints an EWG for each of the technical topics chosen. This reviews differences in requirements between the three regions and begins development of scientific consensus. The membership of EWGs is not 'fixed'. Each party nominates a Topic Leader (and, often, a Deputy Topic Leader) as the contact point. Observers to ICH, pharmacopoeial authorities and representatives from the nonprescription medicinal product industry and the generic industry may be invited to join relevant EWGs.

An EWG can only meet officially (in its ICH capacity) if at least one nominated expert from each of the six ICH co-sponsors is present.

The harmonisation process

A stepwise process has been developed to track the progress of each guideline during the harmonisation process. This identifies the work remaining to reach a defined endpoint. The process is primarily applicable to the development of harmonised tripartite guidelines or other statements of position.

The initial impetus to select a harmonisation topic is the production of a concept paper by one of the six ICH parties or an EWG. The concept paper outlines areas of difference and where harmonisation could be achieved. A decision on proceeding with the harmonisation process is then taken by the ICH Steering Committee.

Step 1

A six-party EWG is appointed for the topic, with one of the Topic Leaders appointed as topic rapporteur. Preliminary discussions on the topic between EWG members result in a first draft document prepared by the rapporteur. The document may be a draft guideline, a policy statement, a recommendation or a 'Points to Consider' document. Successive drafts are prepared by the experts until scientific consensus is achieved. The draft document is then passed to the Steering Committee.

Step 2

The draft is 'signed off' by each of the six parties to the Steering Committee. Regulatory authorities in the three regions are sent the Step 2 draft and formal consultation is undertaken in each region. A period of 6 months is usually allowed for comments to be submitted.

Step 3

A Regulatory Rapporteur is appointed from one of the three regulatory authorities. This Rapporteur collates and analyses the comments and ensures that all regulatory bodies are aware of them. If necessary, the Rapporteur also amends the Step 2 draft document.

If it is clear that there has been a move away from scientific consensus during the consultation process, the regulatory authorities may decide to send out the amended draft for further comments.

If consensus appears likely as a result of the consultation process, a final draft is prepared by the Regulatory Rapporteur, which must then be agreed with the other five parties' representatives. With this achieved, a final draft is sent to the relevant ICH EWG. If the EWG is happy with the document, it is 'signed off' by the experts from the six parties, after which the document is referred to the ICH Steering Committee for adoption.

Step 4

There has to be agreement on the composition of the final draft by the Steering Committee. If achieved, it is 'signed off' by the regulatory bodies in the EU, the USA and Japan, and they recommend the three regulatory bodies to incorporate the text within existing legislation in their regions.

Step 5

Step 5 is achieved when the Step 4 document has been assimilated into the regional or national regulations or other appropriate action has been taken.

ICH topics and guidelines

The content of an MAA is divided into topics covering quality, safety and efficacy. ICH topics are similarly divided and coded as 'Q', 'S' and 'E' topics; a fourth category covers multidisciplinary ('M') topics:

- 'Quality' topics cover chemical and pharmaceutical quality assurance.
- 'Safety' topics relate to *in vitro* and *in vivo* preclinical studies.
- 'Efficacy' topics relate to clinical studies in human subjects.
- 'Multidisciplinary' topics are those that do not fit into one of the above categories.

The guidelines which have been promulgated through the ICH process are listed in Table 13.3.

Table 13.3 ICH guidelines

General class	ICH code	Guideline title
Quality topics		
Stability	Q1	
	Q1A (R2)	Stability Testing of New Drugs and Products (second revision)
	Q1B	Photo-Stability Testing
	Q1C	Stability Testing: New Formulations
	Q1D	Bracketing and Matrixing Designs for Stability Testing of Drug Substances and Drug Products
	Q1E	Evaluation of Stability Data
	Q1F	Stability Data Package for Registration in Climatic Zones III and IV
Analytical validation	Q2	
	Q2A	Definitions and Terminology
	Q2B	Methodology
Impurities	Q3	
	Q3A (R)	Impurities in New Drug Substances (first revision)
	Q3B (R)	Impurities in Dosage Forms (first revision)
	Q3C	Impurities: Residual Solvents
Pharmacopoieas	Q4	Pharmacopoeial Harmonisation
Biotechnological quality	Q5	
	Q5A	Viral Safety Evaluation
	Q5B	Genetic Stability
	Q5C	Stability of Products
	Q5D	Cell Substrates
Specifications	Q6	
	Q6A	Chemical Substances
	Q6B	Biotechnological Substances
GMP	Q7	
	Q7A	GMP for Active Pharmaceutical Ingredients
Safety topics		
Carcinogenicity	S1	
	S1A	Need for Carcinogenicity Studies
	S1B	Testing for Carcinogenicity
	S1C	Dose Selection
Genotoxicity	S2	
	S2A	Specific Aspects of Regulatory Tests
	S2B	Standard Battery of Tests
Kinetics	S3	
	S3A	Toxicokinetics
	S3B	Pharmacokinetics
Toxicity	S4	
	S4A	Duration of Chronic Toxicity Testing in Animals (Rodent and Non Rodent Toxicity Testing)
Reproductive toxicity	S5	
	S5A	Toxicity to Reproduction
	S5B	Male Fertility (Maintenance)

continued

Table 13.3 ICH guidelines (*cont.*)

General class	ICH code	Guideline title
Biotechnological safety	S6	Safety Studies for Biotechnological Products
Pharmacology	S7	
	S7A	Safety Pharmacology Studies for Human Pharmaceuticals
	S7B	Safety Pharmacology Studies for Delayed Ventricular Repolarization
Efficacy topics		
Exposure	E1	The Extent of Population Exposure to Assess Clinical Safety
Clinical safety	E2	
	E2A	Definitions and Standards for Expedited Reporting
	E2B (M)	Data Elements for Transmission of ADR Reports (Maintenance) including M2 (see below)
	E2C	Periodic Safety Update Reports
Study reports	E3	Clinical Study Reports: Structure and Content
Dose response	E4	Dose–Response Information to Support Drug Registration
Ethnic factors	E5	Ethnic Factors in the Acceptability of Foreign Clinical Data
GCP	E6	Good Clinical Practice
Special populations	E7	Clinical Trials in Special Populations – Geriatrics
Clinical trial design	E8	General Considerations
	E9	Statistical Considerations
	E10	Choice of Control Group
	E11	Clinical Investigation of Medicinal Products in the Paediatric Population
Therapeutic categories	E12	
	E12A	Clinical Trials on Antihypertensives
Multidisciplinary topics		
	M1	Medical terminology
	M2	Electronic Standards for Transmission of Regulatory Information (ESTRI)
	M3	Timing of Pre-clinical Studies in Relation to Clinical Trials
	M4	The Common Technical Document

The US Food and Drug Administration

The US Food and Drug Administration (FDA) is the largest regulatory agency in the world, covering a vast array of products and responsibilities. Its primary role is the protection of public health by:

- Promoting the public health by promptly and efficiently reviewing clinical research and taking appropriate action on the marketing of regulated products in a timely manner.
- With respect to such products, protecting the public health by ensuring that foods are safe, wholesome, sanitary and properly labelled; that human and veterinary drugs are safe and effective; that there is reasonable assurance of the safety and effectiveness of devices intended

for human use; that cosmetics are safe and properly labelled; and that public health and safety are protected from electronic product radiation.
- Participating through appropriate processes with representatives of other countries to reduce the burden of regulation, harmonise regulatory requirements, and achieve appropriate reciprocal arrangements.
- As determined to be appropriate by the Secretary, carrying out paragraphs (1) through (3) in consultation with experts in science, medicine and public health, and in co-operation with consumers, users, manufacturers, importers, packers, distributors and retailers of regulated products.

It achieves these objectives through a number of Centers:

- Center for Biologics Evaluation and Research (CBER)
- Center for Devices and Radiological Health (CDRH)
- Center for Drug Evaluation and Research (CDER)
- Center for Food Safety and Applied Nutrition (CFSAN)
- Center for Veterinary Medicine (CVM)
- National Center for Toxicological Research (NCTR)
- Office of the Commissioner (OC)
- Office of Regulatory Affairs (ORA).

It also has two affiliated organisations:

- Joint Institute for Food Safety and Applied Nutrition
- National Center for Food Safety and Technology.

The FDA is one of the USA's oldest consumer protection agencies. Its approximately 9000 employees monitor the manufacture, importation, transport, storage and sale of about $1000 billion worth of products each year. The FDA is an agency within the Public Health Service, which in turn is a part of the Department of Health and Human Services (DHHS). It is headed by a Commissioner who is appointed by the DHHS. Many of the offices for the FDA are located in and around the Washington, DC area.

The FDA is a public health agency and has about 1100 investigators and inspectors who monitor the country's almost 95 000 FDA-regulated businesses. These employees are located in district and local offices in 157 cities across the country.

The two most important centers for regulation of pharmaceuticals are the CDER and the CBER.

CDER

The Center for Drug Evaluation and Research (CDER) is the largest of the FDA's Centers, employing about 1800 people. In 2002, it approved 78 new medicinal products, including 17 new chemical entities. It also approved more than 150 new or extended uses of already approved medicinal products (line extensions). It has also been active in removing prescription-only medicines to nonprescription status, making safer and longer-established medicines more readily available. Like other FDA Centers, it has been required to prepare for attacks with chemical, biological and nuclear weapons and to approve countermeasures being tested in animals when human safety and efficacy studies are not practicable.

Also in 2002, CDER undertook a review of the standards of Good Manufacturing Practice currently in place in the pharmaceutical industry. In particular, the review aimed to ensure that the regulatory review programme and the inspection programme for manufacturing sites are effectively co-ordinated without impeding innovation in pharmaceutical manufacturing.

CBER

The Center for Biologics Evaluation and Research (CBER) regulates biological products. Current authority for this responsibility resides in Section 351 of the Public Health Service Act and in specific sections of the Food Drug and Cosmetic Act. The mission of CBER is to protect and enhance the public health through the regulation of biological and related products including blood, vaccines, tissue, allergenics and biological therapeutics.

CBER is responsible for ensuring:

- the safety of the USA's blood supply and the products derived from it
- the production and approval of safe and effective childhood vaccines, including any future AIDS vaccines
- the proper oversight of human tissue for transplantation
- an adequate and safe supply of allergenic materials and antitoxins
- the safety and efficacy of biological therapeutics, including biotechnology-derived products used to treat diseases such as cancer and AIDS.

Biologicals, in contrast to drugs that are chemically synthesised, are derived from humans, animals and microorganisms. As a result, they are complex mixtures that are not easily identified or characterised, and many biologicals are manufactured using biotechnology.

CBER's review of new biological products, and of new indications for already approved products, requires the evaluation of scientific and clinical data to determine whether the product meets CBER's standards for approval. After a thorough assessment of the data, CBER makes a decision based on the risk/benefit for the intended population and the product's intended use.

The World Health Organization

The World Health Organization (WHO) is not a regulatory authority itself, in that it does not assess nor approve medicinal products for supply in individual countries. However, it has been a strong advocate of trying to ensure that all people in its 193 member countries (which comprise almost all countries around the globe) have access to high-quality, safe and effective medicinal products.

The WHO is divided into six Regional Offices whose member states are listed in Appendix 3. Its headquarters are in Geneva, Switzerland, and the work involving monitoring the supply of medicines is carried out by the Department of Essential Drugs and Medicines Policy, also based in Geneva. Its work has been defined by a policy document, *WHO Medicines Strategy: Framework for Action in Essential Drugs and Medicines Policy 2000–2003*, published in 2000.

WHO's strategy is concerned with the supply of essential medicines to the estimated one-third of the world's population who do not have access to them, a figure which it estimates rises to almost one-half in the poorest parts of Africa and Asia. It is also concerned with the fact that, even when such medicines are available, many of them may be of very poor quality or even counterfeit, often owing to the weak regulation that applies in many poorer countries. When essential medicines are available, WHO also tries to educate suppliers and users on their rational use. Too often, it believes, overuse of antibiotics, inappropriate use of injection formulations, and the incorrect use of all drugs by patients aggravate the situation already created by poor regulation.

It has been estimated that fewer than 20% of its Member States have a well-developed drug regulation system. Conversely, almost one-third of its member countries either have no drug regulatory authority or, if one exists, its operational activity is well below that required to be effective.

Some problem areas

In some countries, the legislation covering medicinal products and medical devices is not comprehensive. It may not cover all products for which medicinal claims are made, so allowing certain classes of product to bypass the regulatory controls. Equally, although in most well-developed countries legislation covers manufacture, distribution, importation, dispensing, and advertising and promotion, some of these functions may be exempt from controls in other countries.

A further problem is that the regulatory authority may be responsible not only for the assessment of medicinal products but also for manufacture of medicinal products within the country, for procurement from local manufacturers and from other countries, and for distribution. As a result, conflicts of interest can arise that may lead to the supply of substandard products and services.

Additionally, any lack of consistency between the registration of products manufactured by the state and those manufactured by private enterprises inevitably leads to poorer-quality products being supplied locally. This is illustrated by some countries exempting state-manufactured products from registration, whilst those made by private enterprises are subject to full legislative controls. If the state also has a financial interest in the manufacture of medicinal products for export, the failure to implement full manufacturing controls can lead to distribution of substandard products.

One of the most important aspects for organisations wishing to register their products in less-developed countries is that the regulatory assessment process should be transparent. The regulatory authority should have available standard operating procedures (SOPs) for its administrative processes and checklists for inspections so that manufacturers know the criteria being employed for assessment. Without such publicly available guidelines, the potential for corrupt practices is all the greater.

By definition, all regulatory authorities are government bodies. One of the main difficulties facing poorer countries is the recruitment, retention and payment of well-qualified staff who have a strong desire for and the integrity to implement the supply of safe and effective medicinal products within their country. Governments worldwide are notorious for their relatively poor salaries, even in the relatively few countries in which the regulatory authority is self-financing. In many countries, the fees charged by the authority for the assessment of MAAs rarely cover the cost of an effective assessment. The shortfall in income has to be derived from general taxation and, unless a government deems the supply of safe and effective medicines a high priority, such funding is usually absent or inadequate. Further complications arise in those countries where the salaries of employees and those working on the expert committees carrying out the assessments are linked to the fee income of the authority. This can clearly have an influence on the regulatory decisions by assessors.

Appendix 1

EU regulatory authorities

Austria
Federal Ministry of Health
BfArM
Stubenring 1
1010 Vienna
Tel: + 43 (1) 711 72-0
Fax: + 43 (1) 711 72-4830
www.bmg.gv.at

Belgium
Pharmaceutical Inspectorate
Cité Administrative de l'Etat
Quartier Vésale
Rue Montagne de l'Oratoire 20
B-1010 Brussels
Tel: + 32 (2) 227 56 10
Fax: + 32 (2) 227 55 55
www.afgip.fgov.be

Cyprus
Ministry of Health (Cyprus)
7 Larnacos Avenue
Lefkosia
Nicosia CY-1475
Tel: +357 22 407 105
Fax: +357 22 407 149

Czech Republic
State Institute for Drug Control
Srobarova 48
100 41 Prague 10
Tel: +420 272 185 111
Fax: +420 271 732 377
www.sukl.cz

Denmark
Danish Medicines Agency
378 Frederikssundsvej
DK-2700 Broenshoej
Tel: +45 44 88 9111
Fax: +45 44 91 7373
www.laegemiddelstyrelsen.dk/index_en.htm

Estonia
State Agency for Medicines
Ravila 19
50411 Tartu
Tel: +372 7 37 41 40
Fax: +372 7 37 41 42
www.sam.ee

European Agency for the Evaluation of Medicinal Products
7 Westferry Circus
Canary Wharf
London E14 4HB
England
Tel: +44 (20) 8418 8400
Fax: +44 (20) 8418 8416
www.emea.eu.int

European Commission
DG III/E/3 'Pharmaceutical products'
European Commission
Rue de la Loi, 200
B-1049 Brussels
Tel: +32 (2) 296 09 41
Fax: +32 (2) 296 15 20
www.pharmacos.eudra.org

Finland
National Agency for Medicines
Department of General Affairs
Siltasaarenkatu 18
PO Box 278
FI-00531 Helsinki
Tel: + 358 (9) 396 72
Fax: + 358 (9) 714 469
www.nam.fi/english/index.html

France
Agence du Medicament
Direction of Drug Evaluation
143-147 Boulevard Anatole France
F-93285 Saint-Denis Cedex
Tel: +33 1 (48) 13 20 00
Fax: +33 1 (48) 13 20 98
www.agmed.sante.gouv.fr

Germany
Federal Institute for Drugs and Medical Devices (BfArM)
Federal Health Office
Seestrasse 10
D-13353 Berlin
Tel: + 49 (30) 45 48 30
Fax: + 49 (30) 45 48 32 07
www.bfarm.de

Greece
National Drugs Organization (EOF)
Av Mesogion 284
155 62 Holargos
Athens
Tel: + 30 (1) 654 7004
Fax: + 30 (1) 654 5535
www.eof.gr

Hungary
National Institute of Pharmacy
Zrinyo str. 3
H-1051 Budapest
Tel: +36 (1) 215 8977
Fax: +36 (1) 266 1001
www.ogyi.hu

Ireland
Irish Medicines Board
Block A, Earlsfort Centre
Earlsfort Terrace
Dublin 2
Tel: + 353 (1) 676 4971-7
Fax: + 353 (1) 676 7836
www.imb.ie

Italy
Drugs Evaluation and Pharmacovigilance Department
Ministry of Health
Viale della Civilta Romana 7
00144 Rome
Tel: + 39 (6) 59 94 32 21
Fax: + 39 (6) 59 94 33 65
www.sanita.it/farmaci

Latvia
State Agency of Medicines
15 Jersikas Street
Riga LV-1003
Tel: +371 707 8424
Fax: +371 707 8428
www.vza.gov.lv

Lithuania
State Medicines Control Agency
14 Traku Street
LT-2001 Vilnius
Tel: +370 37 22 28 23
Fax: +370 37 22 28 23
www.vvkt.lt

Luxembourg
Ministry of Health
Division of Pharmacy and Drugs
10 rue CM Spoo
L-2546 Luxembourg
Tel: +352 478 5590/
+352 478 5593
Fax: +352 22 44 58
www.ms.etat.lu

Malta
Medicines Regulatory Unit
198 Rue d'Argens
Gzira GZR 03
Tel: +356 2343 9000
Fax: +356 2343 9161

Netherlands
Medicines Evaluation Board
Sir W. Churchilllaan 362
PO Box 3008
2280 Rijswijk
Tel: + 31 (70) 340 78 14
Fax: + 31 (70) 340 51 55
www.ebg-meb.nl

Poland
Office for Registration of Medicinal Products, Medical Devices, and Biocides
30/34 Chelmska Street
PL-00-725 Warsaw
Tel: +48 22 851 43 81
Fax: +48 22 851 52 43
www.urpl.gov.pl

Portugal
Directorate of Medical Services and Health Products
INFARMED
Parque Saude de Lisboa
Av Brasil 53
1700 Lisboa
Tel: + 351 (1) 790 8500
Fax: + 351 (1) 795 9116
www.infarmed.pt

Slovak Republic
State Institute for Drug Control
Kvetna 11
825 08 Bratislava
Tel: +421 2 50701 111
Fax: +421 2 55 56 41 27
www.sukl.sk

Slovenia
Agency for Medicinal Products
Kersinikova UL.2
SI-1000
Ljubljana
Tel: +386 (1) 478 6243
Fax: +386 (1) 478 6260
www.gov.si/mz/ang/organivsestavi2.html

Spain
Ministry of Health and Consumer Affairs
Directorate General for Pharmacy and Healthcare Products
Paseo del Prado 18-20
E-28014 Madrid
Tel: + 34 (1) 596 1000
Fax: + 34 (1) 596 1547/1548/4069
www.msc.es/agemed

Sweden
Medical Products Agency
PO Box 26
S-751 03 Uppsala
Tel: + 46 (18) 17 4600
Fax: + 46 (18) 54 8566
www.mpa.se/eng

United Kingdom
Medicines and Healthcare products Regulatory Agency, Market Towers
1 Nine Elms Lane
London
SW8 5NQ
Tel: + 44 (20) 7084 2000
Fax: + 44 (20) 7084 2353
www.mhra.gov.uk

Appendix 2

World Medical Association Declaration of Helsinki

Ethical Principles for Medical Research Involving Human Subjects

Adopted by the 18th WMA General Assembly Helsinki, Finland, June 1964, and amended by 29th WMA General Assembly, Tokyo, Japan, October 1975; 35th WMA General Assembly, Venice, Italy, October 1983; 41st WMA General Assembly, Hong Kong, September 1989; 48th WMA General Assembly, Somerset West, Republic of South Africa, October 1996; and the 52nd WMA General Assembly, Edinburgh, Scotland, October 2000. Note of Clarification on Paragraph 29 added by the WMA General Assembly, Washington 2002.

A. Introduction

1. The World Medical Association has developed the Declaration of Helsinki as a statement of ethical principles to provide guidance to physicians and other participants in medical research involving human subjects. Medical research involving human subjects includes research on identifiable human material or identifiable data.
2. It is the duty of the physician to promote and safeguard the health of the people. The physician's knowledge and conscience are dedicated to the fulfilment of this duty.
3. The Declaration of Geneva of the World Medical Association binds the physician with the words, 'The health of my patient will be my first consideration,' and the International Code of Medical Ethics declares that, 'A physician shall act only in the patient's interest when providing medical care which might have the effect of weakening the physical and mental condition of the patient.'
4. Medical progress is based on research which ultimately must rest in part of experimentation involving human subjects.
5. In medical research on human subjects, considerations related to the well-being of the human subject should take precedence over the interests of science and society.
6. The primary purpose of medical research involving human subjects is to improve the prophylactic, diagnostic and therapeutic procedures and

the understanding of the aetiology and pathogenesis of disease. Even the best proven prophylactic, diagnostic and therapeutic methods must continuously be challenged through research for their effectiveness, efficiency accessibility, and quality.

7. In current medical practice and in medical research, most prophylactic, diagnostic and therapeutic procedures involve risks and burdens.
8. Medical research is subject to ethical standards that promote respect for all human beings and protect their health and rights. Some research populations are vulnerable and need special protection. The particular needs of the economically and medically disadvantaged must be recognized. Special attention is also required for those who cannot give or refuse consent for themselves, for those who may be subject to giving consent under duress, for those who will not benefit personally from the research and for those whom the research is combined with care.
9. Research investigators should be aware of the ethical, legal, and regulatory requirements for research on human subjects in their own countries as well as applicable international requirements. No national ethical, legal, or regulatory requirement should be allowed to reduce or eliminate any of the protections for human subjects set forth in this Declaration.

B. Basic Principles for All Medical Research

10. It is the duty of the physician in medical research to protect the life, health, privacy, and dignity of the human subject.
11. Medical research involving human subjects must conform to generally accepted scientific principles, be based on a thorough knowledge of the scientific literature, other relevant sources of information, and on adequate laboratory and, where appropriate, animal experimentation.
12. Appropriate caution must be exercised in the conduct of research which may affect the environment, and the welfare of animals used for research must be respected.
13. The design and performance of each experimental procedure involving human subjects should be clearly formulated in an experimental protocol. This protocol should be submitted for consideration, comment, guidance and, where appropriate, approval to a specially appointed ethical review committee, which must be independent of the investigator, the sponsor or any other kind of undue influence. This independent committee should be in conformity with the laws and regulations of the country in which the research experiment is performed. The committee has the right to monitor ongoing trials. The researcher has the obligation to provide monitoring information to the committee, especially any serious adverse events. The researcher should also submit to the committee, for review, information regarding funding, sponsors, institutional affiliations, other potential conflicts of interest and incentives for subjects.

14. The research protocol should always contain a statement of the ethical considerations involved and should indicate that there is compliance with the principles enunciated in this Declaration.
15. Medical research involving human subjects should be conducted only by scientifically qualified persons and under the supervision of a clinically competent medical person. The responsibility for the human subject must always rest with a medically qualified person and never rest on the subject of the research, even though the subject has given consent.
16. Every medical research project involving human subjects should be preceded by careful assessment of predictable risks and burdens in comparison with foreseeable benefits to the subject or to others. This does not preclude the participation of healthy volunteers in medical research. The design of all studies should be publicly available.
17. Physicians should abstain from engaging research projects involving human subjects unless they are confident that the risks involved have been adequately assessed and can be satisfactorily managed. Physicians should cease any investigation if the risks are found to outweigh the potential benefits or if there is conclusive proof of positive and beneficial results.
18. Medical research involving human subjects should only be conducted if the importance of the object outweighs the inherent risks and burdens to the subject. This is especially important when the human subjects are healthy volunteers.
19. Medical research is only justified if there is a reasonable likelihood that the populations in which the research is carried out stand to benefit from the results of the research.
20. The subjects must be volunteers and informed participants in the research project.
21. The right of research subjects to safeguard their integrity must always be respected. Every precaution should be taken to respect the privacy of the subject, the confidentiality of the patient's information and to minimize the impact of the study on the subject's physical and mental integrity and on the personality of the subject.
22. In any research on human beings, each potential subject must be adequately informed of the aims, methods, sources of funding, any possible conflicts of interest, institutional affiliations of the researcher, the anticipated benefits and potential risks of the study and the discomfort it might entail. The subject should be informed of the right to abstain from participation in the study or to withdraw consent to participate at any time without reprisal. After ensuring that the subject has understood the information, the physician should then obtain the subject's freely-given informed consent, preferably in writing. If the consent cannot be obtained in writing, the non-written consent must be formally documented and witnessed.
23. When obtaining informed consent for the research project the physician should be particularly cautious if the subject is in a dependent

relationship with the physician or may consent under duress. In that case the informed consent should be obtained by a well-informed physician who is not engaged in the investigation and who is completely independent of this relationship.

24. For a research subject who is legally incompetent, physically or mentally incapable of giving consent or is a legally incompetent minor, the investigator must obtain informed consent from the legally authorized representative in accordance with applicable law. These groups should not be included in research unless the research is necessary to promote the health of the population represented and this research cannot instead be performed on legally competent persons.

25. When a subject deemed legally incompetent, such as a minor child, is able to give assent to decisions about participation in research, the investigator must obtain that assent in addition to the consent of the legally authorized representative.

26. Research on individuals from whom it is not possible to obtain consent, including proxy or advance consent, should be done only if the physical/mental condition that prevents obtaining informed consent is a necessary characteristic of the research population. The specific reasons for involving research subjects with a condition that renders them unable to give informed consent should be stated in the experimental protocol for consideration and approval of the review committee. The protocol should state that consent to remain in the research should be obtained as soon as possible from the individual or legally authorized surrogate.

27. Both authors and publishers have ethical obligations. In publication of the results of research, the investigators are obliged to preserve the accuracy of the results. Negative as well as positive results should be published or otherwise publicly available. Sources of funding, institutional affiliation, and any possible conflicts of interest should be declared in the publication. Reports of experimentation not in accordance with the principles laid down in the Declaration should not be accepted for publication.

C. Additional Principles for Medical Research Combined with Medical Care

28. The physician may combine medical research with medical care, only to the extent that the research is justified by its potential prophylactic, diagnostic, or therapeutic value. When medical research is combined with medical care, additional standards apply to protect the patients who are research subjects.

29. The benefits, risks, burdens and effectiveness of a new method should be tested against those of the best current prophylactic, diagnostic, and therapeutic methods. This does not exclude the use of placebo, or no treatment, in studies where no proven prophylactic, diagnostic, or therapeutic method exists. (*See endnote**)

30. At the conclusion of the study, every patient entered into the study should be assured of access to the best proven prophylactic, diagnostic, or therapeutic methods identified by the study.
31. The physician should fully inform the patient which aspects of the care are related to the research. The refusal of a patient to participate in a study must never interfere with the patient-physician relationship.
32. In the treatment of a patient, where proven prophylactic, diagnostic, or therapeutic methods do not exist or have been ineffective, the physician, with informed consent from the patient, must be free to use unproven or new prophylactic, diagnostic, or therapeutic measures, if in the physician's judgement it offers hope of saving life, re-establishing health or alleviating suffering. Where possible, these measures should be made the object of research, designed to evaluate their safety and efficacy. In all cases, new information should be recorded and, where appropriate, published. The other relevant guidelines of this Declaration should be followed.

Note of Clarification on Paragraph 29 of the WMA Declaration of Helsinki.
The WMA hereby reaffirms its position that extreme care must be taken in making use of a placebo-controlled trial and that in general this methodology should only be used in the absence of existing proven therapy. However, a placebo-controlled trial may be ethically acceptable, even if the proven therapy is available, under the following circumstances:

- Where for compelling and scientifically sound methodological reasons its use is necessary to determine the efficacy or safety of a prophylactic, diagnostic, or therapeutic method; or
- Where a prophylactic, diagnostic, or therapeutic method is being investigated for a minor condition and the patients who receive placebo will not be subject to any additional risk of serious or irreversible harm.

All other provisions of the Declaration of Helsinki must be adhered to, especially the need for appropriate ethical and scientific review.

Appendix 3

WHO Member States by region

WHO African Region (AFRO)

Algeria	Côte d'Ivoire	Liberia	Senegal
Angola	Democratic Republic of the Congo	Madagascar	Seychelles
Benin	Equatorial Guinea	Malawi	Sierra Leone
Botswana	Eritrea	Mali	South Africa
Burkina Faso	Ethiopia	Mauritania	Swaziland
Burundi	Gabon	Mauritius	Togo
Cameroon	Gambia	Mozambique	Uganda
Cape Verde	Ghana	Namibia	United Republic of Tanzania
Central African Republic	Guinea	Niger	Zambia
Chad	Guinea-Bissau	Nigeria	Zimbabwe
Comoros	Kenya	Rwanda	
Congo	Lesotho	São Tomé and Principe	

WHO Region of the Americas (AMRO/PAHO)

Antigua and Barbuda	Colombia	Guyana	Puerto Rico
Argentina	Costa Rica	Haiti	Saint Kitts and Nevis
Bahamas	Cuba	Honduras	Saint Lucia
Barbados	Dominica	Jamaica	Saint Vincent and the Grenadines
Belize	Dominican Republic	Mexico	Surinam
Bolivia	Ecuador	Nicaragua	Trinidad and Tobago
Brazil	El Salvador	Panama	United States of America
Canada	Grenada	Paraguay	Uruguay
Chile	Guatemala	Peru	Venezuela

WHO Eastern Mediterranean Region (EMRO)

Afghanistan	Iraq	Oman	Syrian Arab Republic
Bahrain	Jordan	Pakistan	Tunisia
Cyprus	Kuwait	Qatar	United Arab Emirates
Djibouti	Lebanon	Saudi Arabia	Yemen
Egypt	Libyan Arab Jamahiriya	Somalia	
Iran (Islamic Republic of)	Morocco	Sudan	

WHO European Region (EURO)

Albania	Finland	Lithuania	Slovenia
Andorra	France	Luxembourg	Spain
Armenia	Georgia	Malta	Sweden
Austria	Germany	Monaco	Switzerland
Azerbaijan	Greece	Netherlands	Tajikistan
Belarus	Hungary	Norway	The former Yugoslav Republic of Macedonia
Belgium	Iceland	Poland	Turkey
Bosnia and Herzegovina	Ireland	Portugal	Turkmenistan
Bulgaria	Israel	Republic of Moldova	Ukraine
Croatia	Italy	Romania	United Kingdom
Czech Republic	Kazakhstan	Russian Federation	Uzbekistan
Denmark	Kyrgyzstan	San Marino	Yugoslavia
Estonia	Latvia	Slovakia	

WHO South-East Asia Region (SEARO)

Bangladesh	India	Myanmar	Thailand
Bhutan	Indonesia	Nepal	
Democratic Republic of Korea	Maldives	Sri Lanka	

WHO Western Pacific Region (WPRO)

Australia	Kiribati	New Zealand	Singapore
Brunei Darussalam	Lao People's Democratic Republic	Niue	Solomon Islands
Cambodia	Malaysia	Palau	Tokelau
China	Marshall Islands	Papua New Guinea	Tonga
Cook Islands	Micronesia	Philippines	Tuvalu
Fiji	Mongolia	Republic of Korea	Vanuatu
Japan	Nauru	Samoa	Viet Nam

Index

Notes: page references in *italics* indicate tables. In order to save space in the index the following abbreviations have been used: CPMP, Committee for Proprietary Medicinal Products; EMEA, European Agency for the Evaluation of Medicinal Products; ICH, International Conference on the Harmonisation of the Technical Requirements for the Registration of Pharmaceuticals for Human Use.

aciclovir, *viii*
active implantable medical devices,
   Directive 90/358/EEC, 141
Active Implantable Medical Devices
   Regulations (SI 1995 No. 1671), 141
active pharmaceutical ingredients, quality
   guidelines, 32
active substances, *31*, 34, 38–39
   European Drug Master File procedure, *31*,
      40–42
   new, impurities, 42–43
   quality
      Concept Papers, 33
      impurities, see Impurities
      photo-stability testing, see Photo-
         stability testing
      requirements, *31*, 40
      stability testing, see Stability testing
acute coronary syndrome, treatment, 94
acute respiratory distress syndrome,
   treatment, 94, 95
Ad hoc Working Group on Blood Products,
   187
administrative data (Part 1A), marketing
   authorisation applications, 16
ADROIT Electronically Generated
   Information Service (AEGIS), 169
Adverse Drug Reaction On-line
   Information Tracking (ADROIT), 169
adverse events, 96, *128*
   Directive 2001/20/EC, *119*
   liaison officers' role, 145
   listed, *129*
   medical devices, see Medical devices
   notification, 125–126
   reportable, *12*, *108*, *129*, 132–133, 184
   serious, *100*, *130*
   suspected, 125–126, 132

unexpected, *101*, *119*, 125–126, *130*
unlisted, *131*
see also Local tolerance testing
Adverse Incident Centre, 174–175
advertising controls, 164
Advisory Board on the Registration of
   Homeopathic Products, 18
Agence du Medicament, France, 230
Agency for Medicinal Products, Slovenia,
   231
age of consent, clinical trials participation
   and, 149, 154
   see also Children
AIC investigations, 144
allergic rhinoconjunctivitis, treatment, 93
allopurinol, *vii*
Alzheimer's disease, treatment, 91
amlodipine, 5
ampicillin, *vii*
amyotrophic lateral sclerosis, treatment,
   94
analytical procedures validation
   definitions and terminology, 50–51
   methodology, 48–50
   quality guidelines, *32*, 33, 222
angina, treatment, 91
animal studies, 62, 63–66
   autopsies, 63, 73, 83
   criteria, 68
   husbandry, 65
   in vitro models, replacement by, 60
   pharmacotoxicological testing, see
      Pharmacotoxicological studies
   see also Carcinogenicity studies
antiarrhythmics, 91
antibacterial medicinal products, 91, 93, 94
anticancer medicinal products, 60, 90
antifungal agents, 94

243

antihypertensives, clinical trials, *91*, *92*, 223
antioxidants, 30
appraisal (of health interventions), NICE, see National Institute for Clinical Excellence (NICE)
Appraisal of New and Existing Technologies: Interim Guidance for Manufacturers and Sponsors, 202, 207
area under the curve (AUC), 78, 80
arterial occlusive disease (peripheral), treatment, 90
asthma
  inhaler systems/devices, see Inhaler systems/devices
  treatment, 91
atorvastatin, 5
audit, 96, 109
Austria, Federal Ministry of Health, 229
auto-immune disorders, 9
autopsies, animal, 63, 73, 83
azacitidine, *187*
azathioprine, *viii*

baseline covariates, adjustment for, 94
beclometasone, *viii*
Belgium, Pharmaceutical Inspectorate, 229
beta interferon, 204
bioavailability, 31, 90
bioequivalence, 31, 90
Biological and Biotechnology Assessment Group, 161
biostatistical issues, 93, 94
biotechnological products
  cancer treatment, 9
  efficacy guidelines, *91*
  preclinical biological safety testing, 85–87
  quality/safety guidelines, 32, 33, 60, 222–223
  screening, 8–9
Biotechnology Working Party, 186, 188
bipolar disorder, treatment, 90
blastocysts, ethics in research, 151
blinding, 97
blood pressure (elevated), see Hypertension
blood products, safety testing, 87
breast cancer, 203
  medicinal products, 60, 90
British National Formulary, 12
British Pharmacopoeia, 166
British Pharmacopoeia Commission, 18
bromelain, *187*
bryostatin-1, *187*
Business Licensing Information Services (BLIS), 169

cancer
  biotechnological agents in treatment of, 9
  breast, see Breast cancer
  ovarian, *203*
  see also Anticancer medicinal products; Carcinogenicity studies
captopril, *viii*
carcinogenicity studies, 81
  biotechnological products, 86
  detection, 71–74
  dose selection, 76–79
  guidelines, 60, 222
  insulin, 62
  need for, 74–76
cardiac failure, treatment, 90, 93
cardiac pacemakers, 141
cardiovascular events, secondary prevention, modified release products, 90
carmustine, *187*
case-control studies, 137
case histories, 136
Case Report Form, 97
case safety reports, 92
case surveillance studies, 137
CE mark, 143
Center for Biologics Evaluation and Research (CBER), 224, 225
Center for Devices and Radiological Health (CDRH), 224
Center for Drug Evaluation and Research (CDER), 224–225
Center for Food Safety and Applied Nutrition (CFSAN), 224
Center for Veterinary Medicine (CVM), 224
Central Office of Research Ethics Committee (COREC), 122
cervical screening, liquid-based, *203*
chemical substances, 222
children
  clinical studies and, 120–121
  ethics, 153–154
  see also Informed consent
  efficacy guidelines, 93, 223
chronic obstructive pulmonary disease (COPD), treatment, 94
cimetidine, *viii*, 5
clinical effectiveness promotion, 197
  see also National Institute for Clinical Excellence (NICE)
clinical practice, 92
clinical safety, data management, 92, 223
clinical studies, 89–126
  children and, see Children
  Clinical Trials Directive 2001/20/EC see Clinical Trials Directive 2001/20/EC
  conduct, 123–124
  definitions, 97, 118–*119*
  efficacy
    Concept Papers, 93
    guidelines, 90–*91*, *92*, 223

Points to Consider, 94–95
ethics, *see* Ethics
financial inducements, 149–150
Good Clinical Practice guidelines, *see* Good Clinical Practice
investigators, *see* Investigators
medicinal product development, 10–11
  see also Medicinal products
protocols, *see* Protocols
safety reporting, 105–106
screening, 62
sponsors, *see* Sponsors
statistical principles, 92
terms, 96–*102*
Clinical Trial Certificate, 10–11
Clinical Trial Exemption Certificate, 10
Clinical Trial Exemption scheme, 161
Clinical Trials Directive 2001/20/EC, 112–126
  conduct of trials, 123–124
  definitions, 118–*119*
  ethics committees, *see* Ethics committees
  informed consent, *see* Informed consent
  investigational medicinal products, 124–125
  main points, 115–117
  minors, 120–121
  objectives, 114–115
  reasons for legislation, 114
  scope, 117–120
  subjects, protection of, 120
  see also Clinical studies
Clinical Trials Unit, Medicines and Healthcare products Regulatory Agency (MHRA), 161
cloning techniques, 152–153
clopidogrel, *21*
clotrimazole, *viii*
colistemethate sodium, *187*
Collaborating Centre for International Drug Monitoring, 185
Committee for Human Medicinal Products (CHMP), 28, 132, 140, 183
  evaluation, 189–190
  see also Committee for Proprietary Medicinal Products (CPMP)
Committee for Orphan Medicinal Products (COMP), 28, 181, 186, 188
Committee for Proprietary Medicinal Products (CPMP), 28, 179, 181
  ad hoc working groups, 188
  centralised procedure, 20
  efficacy
    Concept Papers, 93
    guidelines, 90–*91*
    Points to Consider, 94–95
  Invented Names Review Group, 187–188
  multi-state procedure, 19

pharmacotoxicological studies, *see* Pharmacotoxicological studies
quality
  Concept Papers, *33*
  guidelines, 30–*31*
  see also Committee for Human Medicinal Products (CHMP)
Committee for Veterinary Medicinal Products (CVMP), 20, 28, 29, 179, 181
  quality guidelines, 30–*31*
Committee of Herbal Medicinal Products, 28
Committee on Safety of Devices, 145
Committee on Safety of Drugs, 18
Committee on Safety of Medicines, 18–19, 123
Common Technical Document, 15, 26–27, *223*
Community Code, 27
community pharmacists, 12
Company Core Data Sheet (CCDS), *128*, 136
comparative studies, 212
comparators (product), 97
compensation (subjects and investigators), 107
Competence Development Framework, 167
compliance (in relation to trials), 97
concertation procedure, 19–20
confidentiality, 206
consent
  age of, clinical trials participation and, 149, 154
  informed, *see* Informed consent
consumer protection agencies, 224
contraceptives, steroid, *90*, vii
Contract Research Organisation, 97
control groups, 137, *223*
control groups (in clinical studies), 92
Coordinating Committee, 97
Coordinating Investigator, 97
coronary artery stent development, *203*
coronary heart disease, treatment, *203*
Corporate Services Group, 167
costs
  medicinal product development, 4–5
  NICE submissions, 212, 213
CPMP/115/01, 30
CPMP/180/95, 90
CPMP/372/01, 62
CPMP/602/95 Rev. 3, *94*
CPMP/986/96, 62
CPMP/2330/99, *94*
CPMP/3097/02, *60*, *91*
CPMP/CVMP/QWP/115/95, *30*
CPMP/EWP/18/01, *91*
CPMP/EWP/021/97, *94*, *95*
CPMP/EWP/49/01, *91*
CPMP/EWP/197/99, *94*

CPMP/EWP/205/95, *90*
CPMP/EWP/225/02, *93*
CPMP/EWP/226/02, *93*
CPMP/EWP/234/95, *91*
CPMP/EWP/235/95, *90*
CPMP/EWP/237/95, *91*
CPMP/EWP/238/95, *90*
CPMP/EWP/239/95, *91*
CPMP/EWP/240/95, *91*
CPMP/EWP/280/96, *90*
CPMP/EWP/281/96, *91*
CPMP/EWP/282/02, *90*
CPMP/EWP/462/95, *91*
CPMP/EWP/463/97, *90*
CPMP/EWP/482/99, *94*
CPMP/EWP/504/97, *94*, *95*
CPMP/EWP/512/01, *93*
CPMP/EWP/518/97, *90*
CPMP/EWP/519/98, *90*
CPMP/EWP/520/96, *91*
CPMP/EWP/552/95, *90*
CPMP/EWP/553/95, *91*
CPMP/EWP/555/95, *91*
CPMP/EWP/556/95, *94*, *95*
CPMP/EWP/558/95, *91*
CPMP/EWP/559/95, *91*
CPMP/EWP/560/95, *91*
CPMP/EWP/560/98, *94*
CPMP/EWP/561/98, *90*
CPMP/EWP/562/98, *94*
CPMP/EWP/563/95, *90*
CPMP/EWP/563/98, *90*
CPMP/EWP/565/98, *94*
CPMP/EWP/566/98, *90*
CPMP/EWP/567/98, *90*
CPMP/EWP/570/98, *94*
CPMP/EWP/612/00, *91*
CPMP/EWP/633/02, *91*
CPMP/EWP/707/98, *94*
CPMP/EWP/714/98, *90*
CPMP/EWP/784/97, *94*, *95*
CPMP/EWP/785/97, *94*
CPMP/EWP/788/01, *91*
CPMP/EWP/863/98, *94*
CPMP/EWP/908/99, *94*
CPMP/EWP/967/01, *93*
CPMP/EWP/968/02, *93*
CPMP/EWP/1080/00, *90*
CPMP/EWP/1119/98, *94*
CPMP/EWP/1343/01, *94*
CPMP/EWP/1412/01, *93*
CPMP/EWP/1533/01, *93*
CPMP/EWP/1776/99, *94*
CPMP/EWP/2158/99, *93*
CPMP/EWP/2284/99, *94*
CPMP/EWP/2339/02, *93*
CPMP/EWP/2454/02, *93*
CPMP/EWP/2455/02, *93*
CPMP/EWP/2459/02, *93*
CPMP/EWP/2655/99, *94*
CPMP/EWP/2747/00, *90*
CPMP/EWP/2863/99, *94*
CPMP/EWP/2922/00, *91*
CPMP/EWP/2991/01, *93*
CPMP/EWP/4151/00, *94*
CPMP/EWP/PhVWP/1417/01, *93*
CPMP/EWP/QWP/1401/98, *31*, *90*
CPMP/ICH/135/95, 89–112, *92*
CPMP/ICH/137/95, *92*
CPMP/ICH/138/95, *33*
CPMP/ICH/139/95, *33*
CPMP/ICH/141/95, 71
CPMP/ICH/142/95, *32*, *33*
CPMP/ICH/279/95, *32*, 54–56
CPMP/ICH/280/95, *32*
CPMP/ICH/281/95, *32*
CPMP/ICH/281/96, 48–50
CPMP/ICH/282/95, *32*, *33*, 46–47
CPMP/ICH/283/95, *32*
CPMP/ICH/287/95, *92*
CPMP/ICH/288/95, *92*
CPMP/ICH/289/95, *92*
CPMP/ICH/291/95, *92*
CPMP/ICH/294/95, *32*
CPMP/ICH/295/95, *32*
CPMP/ICH/363/96, *92*
CPMP/ICH/364/96, *92*
CPMP/ICH/365/96, *32*
CPMP/ICH/367/96, *32*
CPMP/ICH/375/95, *92*
CPMP/ICH/377/95, *92*
CPMP/ICH/378/95, *92*
CPMP/ICH/379/95, *92*
CPMP/ICH/380/95, *32*, *33*, 51–54, *51*
CPMP/ICH/381/95, *33*, 50–51
CPMP/ICH/383/95, 76–79
CPMP/ICH/384/95, 79–82
CPMP/ICH/385/95, 66–67
CPMP/ICH/420/02, *33*
CPMP/ICH/421/02, *33*
CPMP/ICH/541/00, *92*
CPMP/ICH/1940/00, *32*
CPMP/ICH/2711/99, *92*
CPMP/ICH/2736/99, *32*
CPMP/ICH/2737/99, *32*
CPMP/ICH/2738/99, *33*
CPMP/ICH/3801/95, 54
CPMP/ICH/4104/00, *32*
CPMP/ICH/4106/00, *32*
CPMP/ICH/4679/02, *92*
CPMP/QWP/054/98, *30*
CPMP/QWP/072/96, *30*
CPMP/QWP/115/95, *30*
CPMP/QWP/122/02, *31*
CPMP/QWP/130/96 Rev. 1, *31*
CPMP/QWP/155/96, *31*
CPMP/QWP/158/01, *30*
CPMP/QWP/158/96, *31*

CPMP/QWP/159/01, *30*
CPMP/QWP/159/96, *31*
CPMP/QWP/227/02, *31*
CPMP/QWP/297/97, *31*
CPMP/QWP/486/95, *31*
CPMP/QWP/556/96, *31*
CPMP/QWP/576/96, *31*
CPMP/QWP/604/96, *30*, *56–57*
CPMP/QWP/609/96, *31*
CPMP/QWP/609/96 Rev. 1, *31*
CPMP/QWP/848/96, *30*
CPMP/QWP/1719/00, *30*
CPMP/QWP/2430/98, *33*
CPMP/QWP/2431/98, *33*
CPMP/QWP/2570/98, *33*
CPMP/QWP/2809/98, *33*
CPMP/QWP/2819/00, *30*
CPMP/QWP/2820/00, *30*
CPMP/QWP/2845/00, *30*
CPMP/QWP/2930/99, *33*
CPMP/QWP/2934/99, *30*
CPMP/QWP/3015/99, *30*
CPMP/QWP/3309/01, *31*
CPMP/QWP/8567/99, *30*
CPMP/SWP/112/98, *60*
CPMP/SWP/160/98, *60*
CPMP/SWP/373/01, *62*
CPMP/SWP/398/01, *60*
CPMP/SWP/465/95, *60*
CPMP/SWP/668/02, *62*
CPMP/SWP/728/95, *60*
CPMP/SWP/781/00, *62*
CPMP/SWP/997/96, *60*
CPMP/SWP/1042/99, *60*, *64–66*
CPMP/SWP/1053/00, *62*
CPMP/SWP/2145/00, *60*
CPMP/SWP/2599/02, *60*
CPMP/SWP/2600/01, *62*
CPMP/SWP/2877/00, *60*
CPMP/SWP/3404/01, *62*
CPMP/SWP/4163/00, *62*
CPMP/SWP/4446/00, *60*
CPMP/SWP/4447/00, *62*
Crohn's disease, management, *94*
cut-off date (data lock-point), *128*
CVMP/271/01, *30*
Cyprus, Ministry of Health, 229
cytokines, 87
cytology, liquid-based, *203*
Czech Republic, State Institute for Drug Control, 229

Danish Medicines Agency, 229
data
  lock-point (cut-off date), *128*
  missing, *94*
Data and Safety Monitoring Board, *98*
Declaration of Geneva, 233
Declaration of Helsinki, 89–92, 148–149, 233–237
Defective Medicines Reporting Centre (DMRC), 165
delayed ventricular repolarization, *223*
Denmark, Danish Medicines Agency, 229
dental care, *203*
Department of Essential Drugs and Medicines Policy, 226
Department of Health (UK), 158, 201
  Health Technology Assessment (HTA) Programme, 207
  Research and Development Directorate, 210
depression, treatment, *90*
dermal tolerance testing, 84
development pharmaceutics/process validation, *31*, *34–35*
Device Alerts, 144–145, 175
Device Bulletins, 175
diabetes mellitus, *90*
diagnostic agents
  biotechnological, 9
  evaluation, *94*
diclofenac, *viii*
direct access, *98*
Directive 65/65/EEC, viii, 19, 20, 23, 216
Directive 75/318/EEC, 20, 23
Directive 75/319/EEC, 19, 20, 23, 127
Directive 75/320/EEC, 19
Directive 87/22/EEC, 19–20, 20
Directive 89/105/EEC, 23
Directive 89/342/EEC, 23
Directive 89/343/EEC, 23
Directive 89/381/EEC, 23
Directive 90/342/EEC, 210
Directive 90/358/EEC, 141
Directive 91/356/EEC, 23
Directive 92/25/EEC, 23
Directive 92/26/EEC, 23
Directive 92/27/EEC, 23
Directive 92/28/EEC, 23
Directive 92/73/EEC, 23
Directive 93/39/EEC, 20, 21, 23
Directive 93/40/EEC, 20
Directive 93/41/EEC, 20, 23
Directive 93/42/EEC, 142
Directive 95/25/EEC, 23
Directive 95/26/EEC, 23
Directive 98/79/EC, 143
Directive 2001/20/EC, *118*, 153–154
Directive 2001/20/EEC, 23
Directive 2001/83/EC, 27
Directive 2001/83/EEC, 23
Directorate of Medical Services and Health Products, Portugal, 231
disability equipment, 176–177
dissemination of information, NICE role, 197, 209

docetaxel, *203*
documentation, *98*
dosage forms, *34–35*
 modified release, *90*, *93*
 quality
  manufacture of finished, *31*
  manufacture of finished forms, *35–36*
  prolonged release oral solid, *56–57*
  stability testing requirements, *54*
 shelf-life, *30*
dose-response information, *92*, *223*
dose selection, *222*
dossier summary, marketing authorisation applications, *7*, *16–18*
double-blind trials, *11*
drug abuse, *128*
drug development, *see* Medicinal products
Drug Information Pharmacists Group, *201*
drug interactions, investigation, *91*
drug reactions, *see* Adverse events
drugs approval tracking system (SIAMED), *193*
Drugs Directorate, Health Canada, *219*
Drugs Evaluation and Pharmacovigilance Department, Italy, *230*
dry powder inhalers, *31*
dyslipoproteinaemia, treatment, *93*
dyspepsia, *204*

EC/ICH/140/95, *74–76*
EC/CPMP/ICH/299/95, *71–74*
eCTD, *192*
Effectiveness Bulletins, *198*
efficacy, *15*, *18*
 clinical studies, *see* Clinical studies
 CPMP guidelines, *see* Committee for Proprietary Medicinal Products (CPMP)
 ICH guidelines, *see* International Conference on the Harmonisation of Technical Requirements for the Registration of Pharmaceuticals for Human Use (ICH)
 see also Pharmacovigilance
eflornithine hydrochloride, *187*
electronic Common Technical Document (eCTD), *192*
Electronic Standards for Transmission of Regulatory Information (ESTRI), *223*
emadine, *21*
emasdistine, *21*
embryos, ethics in research, *150–153*
EMEA/CVMP/134/02, *31*
EMEA/CVMP/598/99, *30*
EMEA/CVMP/814/00, *30*
EMEA/CVMP/815/00, *30*
EMEA/CVMP/961/01, *31*

Enforcement Group, Medicines and Healthcare products Regulatory Agency (MHRA), *165–166*
epileptic disorders, treatment, *90*
epothilone b, *187*
Estonia, State Agency for Medicines, *229*
Ethical Principles for Medical Research Involving Human Subjects, *92*
ethics, *147–154*
 children, research in, *153–154*
 Declaration of Geneva, *233*
 Declaration of Helsinki, *148–149*, *233–237*
 embryonic/fetal tissue research, *150–153*
 ethics committees, *see* Ethics committees
 historical perspectives, *147–148*
 post-authorisation safety studies, company-sponsored, *138*
 stem cell research, *151*, *152–153*
 vulnerable groups, protection of, *149–150*
 see also Ethics committees
Ethics Committee Authority, *122*
ethics committees, *121–123*
 definition, *119*
 independent, *98*, *102–103*
 local, *174*
 multicentre, *174*
 opinions, *100*, *122–123*
ethnic factors
 foreign clinical data acceptability, *92*
 ICH guidelines, *223*
ethylene oxide use, limitations, *30*, *36–37*
EU, *see* European Union (EU)
Eudra Vigilance system, *193*
eugenics, *147–148*
 see also Ethics
European Agency for the Evaluation of Medicinal Products (EMEA), *15*, *29*, *179–193*
 activities, *182–188*, *182*
 administration and support, *191–193*
 biotechnological product approval, *8*
 contact details, *180*, *229*
 efficacy, guidelines, *90–91*
 inspections, *190–191*
 legal framework, *179–180*
 Mission Statement, *182*
 pharmaceutical legislation review, *180–181*
 pharmacotoxicological studies, *see* Pharmacotoxicological studies
 quality
  Concept Papers, *33*
  guidelines, *30–31*
 staff allocations, *191–192*, *192*
 structure, *181–182*
 veterinary medicinal products, evaluation, *189–190*

Index **249**

European and Other International Support unit, 167
European and Regulatory Affairs Group, Medicines and Healthcare products Regulatory Agency (MHRA), 175–176
European Centre for the Validation of Alternative Methods (ECVAM), 9
European Commission
 contact details, 229
 harmonisation process, *218*
 marketing authorisation applications, role in, 25–26
European Council Regulation (EC) No.2309/93, 20
European Drug Master File procedure, *31*, 40–42
 content, information accompanying and documentation, 41
 procedure, 41
European Federation of Pharmaceutical Industries and Associations (EFPIA), *viii*, *218*
European Free Trade Area (EFTA), *219*
European Union (EU)
 birth date (EBD) for authorisations, *128*
 harmonisation process, *218*
 regulatory authorities, 229–231
evaluation (of health interventions), National Institute for Clinical Excellence, *see* National Institute for Clinical Excellence (NICE)
excipients, 44
 development, 34
Executive Support Group, Medicines and Healthcare products Regulatory Agency (MHRA), 166–167
experimental animals, *see* Animal studies
Expert Reports, marketing authorisation applications, 17–18
Expert Working Groups (EWGs), 220
Export Certificates, 165
Export Certificate System (ECS), 169
eyes, local tolerance testing, 83–84

FDA, *see* Food and Drug Administration (FDA)
Federal Institute for Drugs and Medical Devices (BfArM), Germany, 230
Federal Ministry of Health, Austria, 229
Fees, Policy and Litigation Coordination Unit, 167
fertility (maintenance), *222*
fetal monitoring (ultrasound), 175
fetal tissue, 150–153
Finance and Human Resources Division, Medicines and Healthcare products Regulatory Agency (MHRA), 168
financial inducements, clinical trials, 103, 149–150

Finland, National Agency for Medicines, 229
fixed combination medicinal products, *91*
fluconazole, *viii*
flurbiprofen, *viii*
fluticasone, *5*
Food and Drug Administration (FDA), 216, 223–224
 harmonisation process, *218*
 role/objectives, 223–224
forced degradation studies, *55*
France, Agence du Medicament, 230
fumagillin, *187*
fungal infections, treatment, *94*
'Future Systems' legislation, 20, 22

gases (medicinal), *30*
General Practice Research Database, Medicines and Healthcare products Regulatory Agency (MHRA), 168
gene therapy products, safety studies, *60*
genetically modified organisms (GMOs), 29
genetic stability, *222*
genotoxicity, 71, *222*
geriatric populations, *92*, *223*
Germany, Federal Institute for Drugs and Medical Devices (BfArM), 230
glataramer, *204*
Global Harmonisation Task Force (GHTF), 176, 217
globalisation (development of medicinal products/devices), 215–227
 ICH process, *see* International Conference on the Harmonisation of Technical Requirements for the Registration of Pharmaceuticals for Human Use (ICH)
 US Food and Drug Administration, *see* Food and Drug Administration (FDA)
GLP Monitoring Authority, 166
GMP, ICH guidelines, *222*
Good Clinical Practice Compliance Unit, 165
Good Clinical Practice Guideline CPMP/ICH/135/95, 89–112
 definition, *98*
 Independent Ethics Committees, *see* Independent Ethics Committees
 principles, 95–102
Good Laboratory Practice Monitoring Authority, 158
granulocyte-macrophage colony-stimulating factor receptor antagonists, *187*
Greece, National Drugs Organization (EOF), 230

H_2-receptor antagonists, *5*

haematopoietic growth factors, efficacy
  guidelines, 91
  Points to Consider, 94
harmonisation, *see* International Conference on the Harmonisation of Technical Requirements for the Registration of Pharmaceuticals for Human Use (ICH)
Hazard Notices, 144, 174–175
Health Technology Assessment (HTA) Programme, 207
hearing aid technology, 203
heart disease, treatment, 203
heart failure, treatment, efficacy
  Concept Paper, 93
  guidelines, 90
Helicobacter pylori eradication, efficacy
  Points to Consider, 94
hepatic impairment, efficacy Concept Paper, 93
hepatitis B infection
  test kits, 143
  vaccine, 8–9
herbal medicinal products, 30
Herbal Medicinal Products Working Party, 187
hip prostheses/replacement, 203
HIV infection, treatment, 91, 94
homeopathic medicinal products, 22
Homeopathic Registration Scheme, 163
hormone replacement therapy, 94, 95
hormones, safety testing, 87
Hungary, National Institute of Pharmacy, 230
hypertension, treatment, 90, 92

ibuprofen, *viii*
ICH, *see* International Conference on the Harmonisation of Technical Requirements for the Registration of Pharmaceuticals for Human Use (ICH)
ICH E1, Extent of Population Exposure to Assess Clinical Safety, 223
ICH E2, clinical safety, 223
ICH E2A, Definitions and Standards for Expedited Reporting, 223
ICH E2B (M), Data Elements for Transmission of ADR Reports, 223
ICH E2C, Periodic Safety Update Reports, 223
ICH E3, Clinical Study Reports: Structure and Content, 223
ICH E4, Dose–Response Information to Support Drug Registration, 223
ICH E5, Ethnic Factors in the Acceptability of Foreign Clinical Data, 223
ICH E6, Good Clinical Practice, 223
ICH E7, Clinical Trials in Special Populations – Geriatrics, 223
ICH E8, General Considerations, 223
ICH E9, Statistical Considerations, 223
ICH E10, Choice of Control Group, 223
ICH E11, Clinical Investigation of Medicinal Products in the Paediatric Population, 223
ICH E12, therapeutic categories, 223
ICH E12A, Clinical Trials on Antihypertensives, 223
ICH M1, Medical Terminology, 223
ICH M2, Electronic Standards for Transmission of Regulatory Information (ESTRI), 223
ICH M3, Timing of Pre-clinical Studies in Relation to Clinical Trials, 223
ICH M4, Common Technical Document, 223
ICH Q1, Stability, 222
ICH Q1A (R2), Stability Testing of New Drugs and Products, 222
ICH Q1B, Photo-Stability Testing, 222
ICH Q1C, Stability Testing: New Formulations, 222
ICH Q1D, Bracketing and Matrixing Designs for Stability Testing of Drug Substances and Drug Products, 222
ICH Q1E, Evaluation of Stability Data, 222
ICH Q1F, Stability Data Package for Registration in Climatic Zones III and IV, 222
ICH Q2, analytical validation, 222
ICH Q2A, Definitions and Terminology, 222
ICH Q2A, Methodology, 222
ICH Q3, impurities, 222
ICH Q3A (R), Impurities in New Drug Substances, 222
ICH Q3B (R), Impurities in Dosage Forms, 222
ICH Q3C, Impurities: Residual Solvents, 222
ICH Q4, Pharmacopoeial Harmonisation, 222
ICH Q4, pharmacopoeias, 222
ICH Q5, biotechnological quality, 222
ICH Q5A, Viral Safety Evaluation, 222
ICH Q5B, Genetic Stability, 222
ICH Q5C, Stability of Products, 222
ICH Q5D, Cell Substrates, 222
ICH Q6, specifications, 222
ICH Q6A, Chemical Substances, 222
ICH Q6B, Biotechnological Substances, 222
ICH Q7, GMP, 222
ICH Q7A, GMP for Active Pharmaceutical Ingredients, 222
ICH S1, carcinogenicity, 222
ICH S1A, Need for Carcinogenicity Studies, 222

ICH S1B, Testing for Carcinogenicity, *222*
ICH S1C, Dose Selection, *222*
ICH S2, genotoxicity, *222*
ICH S2A, Specific Aspects of Regulatory Tests, *222*
ICH S2B, Standard Battery of Tests, *222*
ICH S3, kinetics, *222*
ICH S3A, Toxicokinetics, *222*
ICH S3B, Pharmacokinetics, *222*
ICH S4, toxicity, *222*
ICH S4A, Duration of Chronic Toxicity Testing in Animals (Rodent and Non Rodent Testing), *222*
ICH S5, reproductive toxicity, *222*
ICH S5A, Toxicity to Reproduction, *222*
ICH S5B, Male Fertility (Maintenance), *222*
ICH S6, biotechnological safety, *223*
ICH S7, pharmacology, *223*
ICH S7A, Safety Pharmacology Studies for Human Pharmaceuticals, *223*
ICH S7B, Safety Pharmacology Studies for Delayed Ventricular Repolarization, *223*
illness, terminal, clinical trials and, 150
immunointerference, 66, 86
Immunologicals Working Party, 190
immunotoxicity, 60
impartial witness, definition, 98
impurities
  active substances, 39
  III/5442/95, 42–43
  guidelines, *32, 33, 222*
  new drugs, 46–47, *222*
incompetent subjects
  Declaration of Helsinki guidelines, 148–149, 236
  see also Vulnerable subjects
incontinence (urinary), treatment, *91*
indemnity, 120
Independent Data Monitoring, 98
Independent Ethics Committees, 98, 102–103
Independent Review Panel for Advertising, 19
Independent Review Panel on the Classification of Borderline Substances, 19
influenza treatment, *204*
information dissemination, NICE role, 197
information leaflets (patient use), 164
Information Management Division, Medicines and Healthcare products Regulatory Agency (MHRA), 169
information technology services
  European Agency for the Evaluation of Medicinal Products (EMEA), 193
  Medicines and Healthcare Products Regulatory Agency (MHRA), 169

informed consent
  clinical trials participation and, 104–105, 120–121, 154
  Declaration of Helsinki guidelines, 235–236
  definition, *99, 119*
infrared spectroscopy, *31*
infusion pumps, 175
inhaler systems/devices, *203*
  efficacy guidelines, *90, 94*
  quality
    Concept Papers, *33*
    guidelines, *30, 31*
inspection, 125
  definition, 99
  Directive 2001/20/EC, *119*
Inspection and Enforcement Division, Medicines and Healthcare products Regulatory Agency (MHRA), 165–166
Institutional Review Board (IRB), *96, 99*
insulin, 9
  carcinogenic potential, 62
  reproductive toxicity, 62
interferon beta, *204*
interferon beta-1a, *21*
interim clinical trial/study report, 99
interleukin 13 chimeric protein, *187*
international birth date (IBD), *129*
International Conference on the Harmonisation of Technical Requirements for the Registration of Pharmaceuticals for Human Use (ICH), 92, 185, 215–227
  conferences, *220*
  co-ordinators, 217
  Expert Working Groups (EWGs), 220
  global harmonisation process, 220–221
  secretariat, *219, 219*
  Steering Committee members/observers, 218–219
  Terms of Reference, 217
  topics and guidelines, 32–33, 221, 222–223
  transparency of process, 219
  see also individual guidelines
intervention studies, *see* Clinical studies
Invented Names Review Group, 187–188
investigational medicinal products, *99, 118,* 124–125
investigators, 103–106
  definition, 99
  selection, 107
Investigator's Brochure, 112
  definition, *99, 118*
  sample title page/table of contents, *113*
in vitro diagnostic (IVD) medical devices, 143
in vitro fertilisation, 152

ionising radiation, 37–38
Irish Medicines Board, 230
irritable bowel syndrome, treatment, *94*
Iscover, *21*
Istin, *5*
Italy, Drugs Evaluation and Pharmacovigilance Department, 230
IVF, 152

Japan
  harmonisation process, *218*
  pharmaceutical controls, 216
Japan Pharmaceutical Manufacturers Association (JPMA), *218*
Joint Institute for Food Safety and Applied Nutrition, 224

kidney disease, *93*
kinetics, *222*

lansoprazole, *5*
Latvia, State Agency of Medicines, 230
legislation (medicines)
  registration options, *see* Registration options
  review, 27–28
levodopa, *viii*
liaison officers, adverse incidents role, 145
licensing applications, *94*
  see also marketing authorisation applications
Licensing Authority, Department of Health, 158
Licensing Division, Medicines and Healthcare products Regulatory Agency (MHRA), 161–163
Lipitor, *5*
Lipostat, *5*
Lithuania, State Medicines Control Agency, 230
liver impairment, *93*
locally applied products, *91*
  see also Local tolerance testing
local research ethics committees (LRECs), 174
local tolerance testing, *60*, 82–84
Losec, *5*
Luxembourg, Ministry of Health, 230

Malta, Medicines Regulatory Unit, 230
marketing authorisation applications, 15
  administrative data (Part 1A), 16
  assessment, *see* European Agency for the Evaluation of Medicinal Products (EMEA); Medicines and Healthcare products Regulatory Agency (MHRA); National Institute for Clinical Excellence (NICE)
  biotechnology products, 9
  centralised procedure, 20–21
    approved products, *21*
    proposed changes, 28
  clinical studies, *see* Clinical studies
  Common Technical Document, 15, 26–27, *223*
  dossier Summary, 7, 16–18
  efficacy issues, *see* Efficacy
  European Commission role, 25–26
  excipients dossier for a medicinal product (III/3196/91), 44
  Expert Reports, 17–18
  holders' responsibilities, 131
  MHRA assessment, 162
  mutual recognition procedure, *see* Mutual recognition procedure
  pharmacotoxicological studies, *see* Pharmacotoxicological studies
  quality issues, *see* Quality
  renewals, 164
  submission, 7, 25
  terms variation, 163–164
  see also Registration options
masking, 97
medical devices
  adverse incidents, 143–145
    liaison officers, role of, 145
    safety warnings, 144–145
    vigilance system, 143–144
  organisations controlling
    EMEA, *see* European Agency for the Evaluation of Medicinal Products (EMEA)
    MHRA, *see* Medicines and Healthcare products Regulatory Agency (MHRA)
    NICE, *see* National Institute for Clinical Excellence (NICE)
  product range, *142*
  regulations, 142
  in vitro diagnostic (IVD), 143
Medical Devices Agency (MDA), 141, 158, 171
Medical devices Directive 93/42/EEC, 142
Medical Devices Regulations (SI 1994 No. 3017), 142
Medical Products Agency, Sweden, 231
medical terminology, *223*
medicinal products
  children, use in, *see* Children
  development process, 3–13, *6*, *8*
    biotechnological screening, 8–9
    clinical studies, 10–11
      see also Clinical studies
    costs, 4–5
    pharmacological screening, 8
    pharmacological testing, preclinical, 9–10
    post-marketing studies, 11–12
    stages, 5–6

fixed combination, *91*
herbal, *30*
homeopathic, 22
impurities, *see* Impurities
investigational, *99*, *118*, *124–125*
organisations controlling
 EMEA, *see* European Agency for the Evaluation of Medicinal Products (EMEA)
 MHRA, *see* Medicines and Healthcare products Regulatory Agency (MHRA)
 NICE, *see* National Institute for Clinical Excellence (NICE)
 WHO role, 225–227
pharmacotoxicological studies, *see* Pharmacotoxicological studies
pharmacovigilance, *see* Pharmacovigilance
registration options, *see* Registration options
top UK, 2002, *5*
veterinary, evaluation, 189–190
vulnerable subjects, *see* Vulnerable subjects
Medicines Act (1968), viii
Medicines Act (1971), 18, 22
Medicines Act Information Letter (MAIL), 167
Medicines and Healthcare products Regulatory Agency (MHRA), 10, 15, 18, 157–169, 202
 advertising controls, 164
 aims/functions, 158–159, 159–160, *159*
 contact details, 231
 Executive Support Group, 166–167
 Finance and Human Resources Division, 168
 General Practice Research Database, 168
 Information Management Division, 169
 Inspection and Enforcement Division, 165–166
 legislative framework, 158
 Licensing Division, 161–163
 Medical Devices Section, 171–177
  European and Regulatory Affairs Group, *173*, *175–176*
  evaluation service, 172, *173*, *176–177*
  functions, 171–172, *173*
  technology and safety, *173*, *174–175*
 Operations Management Team, 160–161
 Post-Licensing Division, 163–164
 responsibilities, *157*
 staffing levels, *160*
Medicines Commission, 18, 19, 123, 159
Medicines Compendium, 17
Medicines Control Agency (MCA), 158, 171
Medicines Evaluation Board, Netherlands, 230

Medicines for Human Use Regulations (1994), 22
Medicines Regulatory Unit, Malta, 230
Memorandum of Understanding, 202
Memorandum of Understanding (MOU), National Institute for Clinical Excellence (NICE), 200
metal catalysts, residue limits, *60*
methodology (clinical studies), *93*
methodology, CPMP, *94*
N-methypyyrolidone, *32*
metronidazole, vii
Microbial Resistance ad hoc group, 190
migraine, treatment, *91*
miltefosine, *187*
Ministry of Health, Cyprus, 229
Ministry of Health, Labor and Welfare, Japan, *218*
Ministry of Health, Luxembourg, 230
Ministry of Health and Consumer Affairs, Spain, 231
minors, *see* Children
Mirapexin, 21
Mission Statement, European Agency for the Evaluation of Medicinal Products (EMEA), *182*
mitotane, *187*
modified release products
 cardiovascular events, secondary prevention, *90*
 efficacy Concept Paper, *93*
 quality guidelines, *30*
monitoring, *100*
monitoring report, *100*
multicentre clinical trials, *118*
multicentre research ethics committees (MRECs), 174
multicentre trials, *100*, 109
multiple sclerosis, treatment, *90*, *204*
multiplicity issues, clinical trials, *94*
'multistate procedure', 19
mutagenicity testing
 biotechnological products, 86
 pharmacotoxicological studies, 69–70
Mutual Recognition Agreements, 176
mutual recognition procedure
 facilitation group, 188
 marketing authorisation applications, 21–22, 162
 proposed changes, 28
myeloablative therapy, *91*
myelosuppressive therapy, *91*
myocardial infarction, treatment, *93*
myristoylated-peptidyl-recombinant scr 1-3 of human complement receptor type i, *187*

National Agency for Medicines, Finland, 229

National Care Standards Commission, 145
National Center for Food Safety and
    Technology, 224
National Center for Toxicological Research
    (NCTR), 224
National Centre for Clinical Audit, 198
National Drugs Organization (EOF),
    Greece, 230
National Electronic Library for Health, 209
National Guidelines Programme, 198
National Health Service, see NHS
National Horizon Scanning Centre, 201
National Institute for Clinical Excellence
    (NICE), 195–214
  appraisal process, 202–208
    Memorandum of Understanding
      (MOU), 200
    uncertain outcomes, 209–210
  guidance documents, 208–209
  initial work programme, 202
    interventions, 203–*204*
  objectives, 195–198
  relationships network, 197–198
  Special Health Authority structure,
    198–200
    Appraisal Group, 199, *199*
    Executive Board, 198–199
    Partners' Council, 199–200
    Secretariat, 200
  sponsors' submissions, proposed data
    requirements, 211–214
  transitional arrangements, 210–211
National Institute of Health Sciences
    (NIHS), Japan, *218*
National Institute of Pharmacy, Hungary,
    230
National Prescribing Centre, 198, 201
Netherlands, Medicines Evaluation Board,
    230
NHS Direct Online, 209
NHS Information Strategy, 197
NHS Research and Development
    Programme, 208
nonclinical studies, *100*
noncompliance (clinical studies), 109
non-genetically modified organisms (non-
    GMOs), environmental risk assessment,
    62
noninterventional trial, *118*, 119
Notice to Applicants, 6
Nuremberg Code, 148

observational cohort studies, 137
ocular tolerance testing, 83–84
Office for Registration of Medicinal
    Products, Medical Devices, and
    Biocides, Poland, 230
Office of Regulatory Affairs (ORA), 224
Office of the Commissioner (OC), 224

olanzapine, *5*
omeprazole, *5*
Operations Management Team, MHRA,
    160–161
opinions (in relation to Independent Ethics
    Committees), *100*
oral contraceptives, vii, *90*
Organisational Matters Group (ORGAM),
    188
orphan medicinal products, 185–186, *187*
orthoclone, *viii*
oseltamivir, *204*
osteoarthritis, treatment, *94*, *95*
osteoporosis (postmenopausal), treatment,
    90
ovarian cancer, *203*
  see also Anticancer medicinal products
overdoses, 134

pacemakers, cardiac, 141
packaging materials, 44–45, 107
paclitaxel, *203*
paediatric populations, see Children
pain, treatment, *91*
Pan-European Regulatory Forum (PERF),
    216
Parallel Import Licensing Scheme, 162
parametric release, quality
  Concept Papers, *33*
  guidelines, *30*
parenteral tolerance testing, 84
Parkinson's disease, treatment, *90*
patient groups, 206
patient information leaflets, 164
payment, clinical trial participation, 103,
    149–150
peptides, pharmokinetics, *93*
Periodic Safety Update Reports, see
    Pharmacovigilance
peripheral arterial occlusive disease,
    treatment, *90*
Pharmaceutical Committee, 19
Pharmaceutical Inspectorate, Belgium,
    229
Pharmaceutical Manufacturers Association
    (IFPMA), *219*
Pharmaceutical Research and
    Manufacturers of America (PhRMA),
    8, 218–*219*
pharmacists, 12
  drug development, involvement in, 3
pharmacodynamic testing, biotechnological
    products, 86
pharmacokinetics, *222*
pharmacology, *223*
Pharmacopoeial Secretariat Group, 166
pharmacopoeias, *222*
pharmacotoxicological studies, 9–10,
    59–87

biotechnological products, preclinical biological safety testing, 85–87
carcinogenicity, *see* Carcinogenicity studies
genotoxicity, 71, *222*
local tolerance testing, *see* Local tolerance testing
mutagenicity, *see* Mutagenicity testing
repeated-dose tissue distribution studies, 66–67
repeated-dose toxicity, 64–66
reproductive toxicity, 62, 67–69, *67, 222*
safety, *see* Safety studies
single-dose toxicity, 60–64
see also Pharmacovigilance; Toxicity studies
pharmacovigilance, 127–140, 163
  adverse drug reaction reporting, *see* Adverse events
  Eudra Vigilance system, 193
  evaluation, post-authorisation, 138–140
    product withdrawal, 140
    risk/benefit assessment, 139
  legal basis and purpose, 127–132
    marketing authorisation holders, responsibilities, 131
    regulatory authority, responsibilities, 131–132
    terminology/definitions, 127, 128–*131*
  Periodic Safety Update Reports, 134–137, 138, 164
    case histories data, 136
    evaluation, 137
    principles, 135
    reporting frequency, 135–136
  post-authorisation safety studies, *129*, 137–138
  special situations, reporting requirements, 133–134
  see also Pharmacotoxicological studies
Pharmacovigilance Working Party, 132, 187, 190
photo-safety testing, 60, 62
photo-stability testing, 32, *222*
  active substances, 54–56
pivotal studies, *94*
placebo, use in medical research, 149
'pluripotent' cells, research, 151, 152–153
Poland, Office for Registration of Medicinal Products, Medical Devices, and Biocides, 230
Policy Group, 166
population exposure, *92*
Portugal, Directorate of Medical Services and Health Products, 231
post-authorisation safety studies
  company-sponsored, 137–138
  definition, *129*

Post-Licensing Division, Medicines and Healthcare products Regulatory Agency (MHRA), 163–164
post-marketing studies, medicinal products development, 11–12
pramipexole, *21*
pravastatin, *5*
preclinical pharmacotoxicological testing, 9–10
preclinical studies, *223*
pregnancy, *93*
  home testing kits, 9, 143
  teratogenic effects reporting, 134
Prescriber's Journal, 198
preservatives, quality guidelines (CPMP/QWP/115/95), *30*
'primitive streak', 151
process validation
  III/847/87, 34–35
  quality guidelines (CPMP/QWP/848/96) (EMEA/CVMP/598/99), *30*
PRODIGY, 197, 198
PRODIGY guidelines, 209
product information management (PIM) project, 192
Product License User System (PLUS), 161, 169
'product profile', 18
product withdrawal, 140
Professional Audit Programme, 198
Prometax, *21*
propranolol, *viii*
proteins, pharmokinetics, efficacy Concept Paper, *93*
protocols
  amendments, clinical studies, 109–111, *110–111*
  definitions, *100, 118*
proton pump inhibitors (PPIs), dyspepsia treatment, *204*
pseudomonas exotoxin, *187*
psoriasis, treatment, *93*

QT interval prolongation, noncardiovascular medicinal products, 62
qualification (of impurities), 43, 47
Qualified Person, pharmacovigilance, 131
qualitative studies, animals, toxicity, 63
quality, 15, 18, 27, 29–57
  active pharmaceutical ingredients, 32
  active substances, *see* Active substances
  analytical procedures validation, *see* Analytical procedures validation
  CPMP guidelines, *see* Committee for Proprietary Medicinal Products (CPMP)
  development pharmaceutics/process validation (III/847/87), 34–35

quality (*cont.*)
  dosage forms, *see* Dosage forms
  ethylene oxide use, limitations (III/9261/90), 36–37
  excipients in MAA dossier for a medicinal product (III/3196/91), 44
  finished product specifications and control tests (III/3324/89), 45–46, *46*
  ICH guidelines, *see* International Conference on the Harmonisation of Technical Requirements for the Registration of Pharmaceuticals for Human Use (ICH)
  impurities, *see* Impurities
  ionising radiation, use in manufacture of medicinal products (III/9109/90), 37–38
  new medicinal products, impurities (CPMP/ICH/282/95), 46–47
  packaging materials, plastic (III/90/90), 44–45
  see also Pharmacovigilance
quality assurance, 106
  definition, *100*
quality control, 106
  definition, *100*
quality of life, assessment, 212
Quality Working Party, 187

radiation, ionising, 37–38
radiopharmaceuticals, quality, Concept Papers, *33*
ramipril, *5*
randomisation, 104
  definition, *100*
ranitidine, *viii*, 5
rapporteurs, 162
  appointment of, 20, 24
Rebif, *21*
rectal tolerance testing, 84
Reference Member State (RMS), 16, 22
reference safety information, Periodic Safety Update Reports, 136
registration options (medicinal products), 15–28
  legislation development, 18–26, 23–24
    pan-European, initial, 19–20
    UK, early, 18–19
    UK/European, existing, 20–24
  marketing authorisation applications, *see* Marketing authorisation applications
Regulation EC 141/2000, orphan medicinal products, *187*
Regulation EC 297/95, *24*
Regulation EC 540/95, *24*
Regulation EC 541/95, *21*, *24*
Regulation EC 542/95, *24*
Regulation EC 1662/95, *24*
Regulation EEC 2309/93, *24*
Regulation No. 2309/93, 20
regulatory authorities
  definition, *100*
  information exchange between, 124
  liaison with, 138
  responsibilities, 131–132
regulatory rapporteur, 221
Remote Access to Marketing Information (RAMA), 169
renal impairment, *93*
repeated-dose tissue distribution studies (CPMP/ICH/385/95), 66–67
repeated dose toxicity, guidelines, *60*
reproductive toxicity, 67–69
  ICH guidelines, *222*
  pharmacotoxicological studies, *62*, 67–69, *67*, *222*
  risk assessment, *62*
research
  children and, 153–154
  protocols, ethical considerations, *see* Ethics
Research and Development Directorate, Department of Health (UK), 210
residual solvents
  ICH guidelines, *222*
  quality guidelines (CPMP/ICH/283/095), *32*
  quality guidelines (CPMP/ICH/1940/00), *32*
  quality guidelines (CPMP/QWP/8567/99), *30*
respiratory distress syndrome (acute), efficacy Points to Consider, *94*, *95*
rheumatoid arthritis, treatment, efficacy Points to Consider, *94*, *95*
rhinoconjunctivitis (allergic), treatment, efficacy Concept Paper, *93*
risk/benefit assessment, 148
  pharmacovigilance evaluation post-authorisation, 139
rivastigmine, *21*
Rules Governing Medicinal Products in the European Union, 6, 29–34, 44

Safety Notices, 145, 175
safety studies, 15, 18
  Discussion/Concept Papers/Points to Consider, *62*
  guidelines, adopted and draft, *60*, *61*
  ICH guidelines, 221, 222–223
  medical devices, *see* Medical devices
  pharmacotoxicological studies, *see* Pharmacotoxicological studies
  photo-safety, *60*, *62*
  post-authorisation, *129*, 137–138
  reporting (in clinical trials), 105–106
  see also Pharmacovigilance
Safety Working Party, 186, 190

salbutamol, *viii*
salmeterol, *5*
schizophrenia, treatment, efficacy guidelines, *91*
Scientific Advice Review Group, 184
screening, cervical, *203*
screening studies, clinical, *62*
Secretary of State for Health, 158
section investigations, 144
sensitivity analysis, 213
Seretide, *5*
Serevent, *5*
severe combined immunodeficiency disease, biotechnological agents in treatment of, *9*
shelf-life (sterile products), quality guidelines (CPMP/QWP/159/96), *31*
SI 1994 No. 3017, 142
SI 1995 No. 1671, 141
SIAMED, 193
sildenafil, *21*
simvastatin, *viii*, *5*
single-dose toxicity, 60–64
skin, local tolerance testing, 84
Slovak Republic, State Institute for Drug Control, 231
Slovenia, Agency for Medicinal Products, 231
sodium cromoglicate, *viii*
solvents, residual
  ICH guidelines, *222*
  quality guidelines (CPMP/ICH/283/095), *32*
  quality guidelines (CPMP/ICH/1940/00), *32*
  quality guidelines (CPMP/QWP/8567/99), *30*
source data, definition, *101*
source documents, definition, *101*
Spain, Ministry of Health and Consumer Affairs, 231
Special Health Authorities, National Institute for Clinical Excellence, *see* National Institute for Clinical Excellence (NICE)
special populations, ICH guidelines, *223*
special situations, reporting requirements, 133–134
sponsor, 106–109, 120
  definition, *101*
  definition, Directive 2001/20/EC, *118*
sponsoring companies, NICE data/evidence required, 205–206, 211–214
sponsor-investigator, definition, *101*
stability testing
  active substances, Guideline CPMP/ICH/380/95, *32*, *33*, 51–54, *51*
  new dosage forms, *see* Dosage forms
  photo-stability, *222*

quality
  Concept Papers, *33*
  guidelines, *30*, *31*, *32*, *33*, *222*
  quality guidelines (CPMP/ICH/421/02), *33*
standard operating procedures (SOPs), *101*, 227
Standards Group, 166
State Agency for Medicines, Estonia, 229
State Agency of Medicines, Latvia, 230
State Institute for Drug Control, Czech Republic, 229
State Institute for Drug Control, Slovak Republic, 231
State Medicines Control Agency, Lithuania, 230
stem cell research, 151, 152–153
sterilisation methods, quality guidelines (CPMP/QWP/054/98), *30*
steroid contraceptives, efficacy guidelines, *90*
storage conditions
  quality guidelines (CPMP/QWP/609/96), *31*
  quality guidelines (CPMP/QWP/609/96 Rev. 1), *31*
stretcher slings, 175
stroke, treatment, *94*
subject identification code, *101*
subject/trial subject
  definition, *101*
  Directive 2001/20/EC, *118*
  protection, 120
sumatriptan, *viii*
Summary of Product Characteristics (SPC), 132, 136
  format, *17*
  marketing authorisation applications, 16–17
superiority, efficacy Points to Consider, *94*
Sweden, Medical Products Agency, 231

tamoxifen, *viii*
taxanes, *203*
Taxol, *203*
Taxotere, *203*
teeth, wisdom, routine extraction, *203*
Telmisartan, *21*
teratogenicity, 134
terminal illness
  clinical trials and, 150
  see also Vulnerable subjects
test procedures/acceptance criteria, *32*
tetrahydrofuran, *32*
thalidomide, 148, vii–viii
therapeutic categories, *223*
thromboembolic disease, treatment, *90*
thymalfasin, 187

Timing of Pre-clinical Studies in Relation to Clinical Trials, 223
tissue distribution studies, repeated-dose, 66–67
tolerance (local) testing, see Local tolerance testing
toxicity studies
  chronic, 75
  ICH guidelines, 222
  pharmacotoxicological studies, 60–64
  repeated-dose, 64–66, 64
  reproductive, 62, 67–69, 67, 222
  single-dose, 60–64
  systematic exposure assessment, 79–82
transferrin, 187
Tritace, 5

ultrasound (fetal monitoring), 175
unblinding (in clinical studies), 104
Unit for Evaluation of Medicinal Products for Human Use, 183
Unit for the Post-authorisation Evaluation of Medicines for Human Use, 183
Unit for the Pre-authorisation Evaluation of Medicines for Human Use, 183
urinary incontinence, treatment, 91
US Food and Drug Administration, see Food and Drug Administration (FDA)

vaccines
  hepatitis B infection, 8–9
  new, 90
  pharmacological and toxicological testing, guidelines, 60
vaginal tolerance testing, 84
venous thromboembolic disease, treatment, 90, 94
ventricular repolarization, delayed, 223
veterinary medical products, evaluation, 189–190
Veterinary Mutual Recognition Facilitation Group, 190
Veterinary Products Committee, 18
Viagra, 21
vigilance system, 143–144
viral safety, 222
vulnerable subjects
  children, see Children
  definition, 102
  informed consent, see Informed consent
  protection, 149–150
    see also Ethics

water (for pharmaceutical use), 30
weight control, drugs used for, 91
well-being (of trial subjects), 102
WHO, see World Health Organization (WHO)
WHO Medicines Strategy: Framework for Action in Essential Drugs and Medicines Policy 2000–2003, 226
wisdom teeth, routine extraction, 203
withdrawal (product), 140
witness, impartial, 98
Working Group on Epidemiology, 188
World Health Organization (WHO), 185
  ICH Steering Committee, observer role, 219
  member states (by region), 239–241
  regulation of medicinal products, role in, 225–227
World Medical Association
  Declaration of Geneva, 233
  Declaration of Helsinki, 89–92, 148–149, 233–237

zanamivir, 204
zidovudine, *viii*
Zocor, 5
Zoton, 5
Zyprexa, 5